YOUR OWN PERFECT MEDICINE

by Martha M. Christy

The *Incredible* Proven Natural Miracle Cure That Medical Science has *Never* Revealed!

Published by

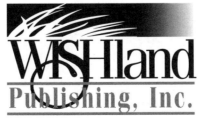

WISHland Publishing, Inc.

P.O. Box 41504
Mesa, Arizona 85274

YOUR OWN PERFECT MEDICINE

by Martha M. Christy

ISBN 0-9632091-1-6
First Printing– May, 1994
Second Printing– August, 1994
Third Printing - October, 1994
Fourth Printing - May, 1996
Fifth Printing - July 1998
Sixth Printing - February 2000

ABOUT THE AUTHOR

Martha Christy is a nutritional and natural health care consultant, medical research writer and editor, and author of the international bestseller *Learn to Control Stress With the Stress Test.* Her other books include *Reconstructing the Real You, Your Body's Best Defense: How pH Balancing Conquers Aging and Disease, Simple Diagnostic Tests You Can Do At Home, Healing Yourself with Homeopathy, Colloidal Silver: The Natural Alternative to Antibiotics, Herbal Grobust: The Natural Way To a Fuller, Firmer Bust Through Herbal Hormone Balancing, MSM: The Super-Supplement of the Decade* and *The Pacific Yew Story: How An Ancient Tree Became a Modern Miracle.*

TABLE OF CONTENTS

CHAPTER ONE

AN AMAZING UNTOLD STORY

There is an extraordinary natural healing substance PRODUCED BY OUR OWN BODIES that modern medical science has proven to be one of the most powerful natural medicines known to man.

Unlike many other natural medical therapies, this method requires no monetary investment or doctors' intervention and can be easily accessed and used at any time.

*The extensive medical research findings on this natural medicine have never been compiled and released to the general public before now, but those who have been fortunate enough to hear about this medicine and use it have found that it can produce often astounding healing **even when all other therapies have failed.***

This book tells of the doctors, medical researchers and the hundreds of other people who have used this extraordinary medicine throughout our century to cure a huge variety of common illnesses and to combat even the most incurable diseases. This is the extraordinary untold story of a natural healing substance so remarkable that it can only be called our own perfect medicine.

M y own experience with this little-known natural medicine began as a result of my search for an answer to many years of serious chronic illnesses that had begun very early in life. Like thousands of people today, I had developed chronic, degenerative disorders that couldn't be helped by conventional medicine and which threatened to permanently destroy my ability to work, function and simply enjoy life.

When I was young, I suffered through the same measles, mumps, chicken pox and colds that everyone else did. And like other children, I played hard, worked hard, and dreamed of the day when I would become a vigorous, emancipated teenager, just like everyone else. But, for me, that particular dream wasn't going to come true.

One beautiful July morning at the age of twelve, I awoke with a start. Suddenly, surprised and frightened, I realized I was lying in a dark red pool of blood that was so large it had soaked through even the thick layers of my mattress. Trembling and weak, I pushed myself up out of bed and felt a horrible, wrenching pain tear through my abdomen.

My worried mother came running in answer to my screams, but after assessing the situation, said there really wasn't much she could do about the pain of my first menstrual period. But what neither she nor I knew at the time, was that what should have been a natural transition to adolescence and menstruating was, for me, going to become a waking nightmare that lasted almost 30 years.

At the onset of each one of my monthly menstrual periods, I would invariably end up either in my doctor's office or at the emergency room of the hospital screaming with pain, bleeding copiously and passing huge clots of blood.

For several months after my 'periods from hell' began, my mother chauffeured me around the city from doctor to doctor with no success until our family doctor finally instituted a monthly regimen of pain killers such as Demerol or Darvon injections and then sent me home with a big, round bottle of full-strength prescription Codeine with which I proceeded to dope myself senseless for the next eight to ten days. This same cycle was repeated every month for almost twenty years.

Throughout adolescence, the simple everyday functions of getting up and going to school were an often monumental and utterly exhausting effort for me. Unlike the rest of my family and friends, I had marked periods of extreme exhaustion. I became extremely susceptible to colds and flu and felt bone-chillingly cold all the time – even in the warmest summer weather.

By the age of fourteen, the effort of combatting severe chronic pain and fatigue while trying to keep up normal activities became impossible. I collapsed and had to be hospitalized and removed from school for several months. But even after a huge battery of medical tests and innumerable visits with doctors and specialists, no one was able to diagnose what was causing my problems.

After many weeks, I returned to school and struggled through the high school years with the aid of generous amounts of codeine and other strong pain killers that my doctor willingly prescribed. But by the time I left home for college, the symptoms of bleeding, exhaustion, pain and digestive problems became so bad that I often was unable to even leave my room or to take part in daily activities.

I kept up the Demerol injections and codeine for many years and added several other new painkillers and drugs which had been developed for menstrual problems to my regimen. But the problems continued unabated and in the ensuing years I developed a myriad of other serious health problems.

During the years from age eighteen to thirty, I was diagnosed with pelvic inflammatory disease, ulcerative colitis, Chron's disease or ileitis (a chronic, painful inflammation of the colon), Chronic Fatigue Syndrome (CFS), Hashimoto's disease (a disorder of the thyroid gland) and mononucleosis.

I had severe chronic kidney infections, two miscarriages, chronic cystitis, severe candida and external yeast infections along with marked adrenal insufficiency and serious chronic ear and sinus infections for which I was prescribed antibiotics on an ongoing basis for several years. Food and chemical allergies also became a big problem. And even though I ate almost nothing because of my extreme food allergies, I actually kept gaining weight, which only added to the discomfort of all the other health disorders I was dealing with.

The bottles of drugs I had taken during this time could have filled a small landfill, but none of my illnesses or disorders had been resolved, and in fact, were more debilitating than ever – it seemed as though I had become nothing more than a walking encyclopedia of disease and the worst part about the entire situation was that no matter how many failed drug therapies I tried, any visit to the doctor's office only resulted in another discouraging failure.

Another big problem was the drug side effects – I felt like a ping-pong ball, bouncing from one drug to another as my doctors kept prescribing more and different drugs to counteract the side effects of the ones I was already taking.

By the time I turned 30, the natural health movement was really picking up speed, and, desperate for any solution, I tried out the Adelle Davis nutrition regimen, mega-vitamin therapy, acupuncture, chiropractic care and every herbal preparation and drug-free natural health therapy that I could find.

Within two years, my chronic cystitis cleared up and the menstrual pain and bleeding markedly decreased. The ulcerative colitis also responded and the sinus infections disappeared. I felt that I was slowly and surely regaining strength and health and even beginning to experience a portion of the energy and vigor that 'normal' healthy people enjoy – and all without drugs. When I conceived my son at 34 and made it through the first trimester without miscarrying I felt as though I'd conquered the final health frontier.

Unfortunately, in my burst of enthusiasm, I underestimated the impact of pregnancy on my understandably frail health, and the birth that I had so carefully prepared for was a near fatal disaster requiring emergency surgery.

And as it turned out, even despite all the illness and pain I'd gone through in the years before the birth, all of it seemed like child's-play after I ran head on into the serious complications of a difficult childbirth.

For months after the birth, I hounded my gynecologist, complaining of unremitting and severe abdominal cramps, cystitis and horribly painful menstrual periods. My natural health treatments would give temporary relief, but mystifyingly, didn't seem to have the same beneficial and lasting effects that they'd had before my pregnancy.

I underwent every conceivable medical test, all of which came back negative, but the problems just didn't go away. My doctor flinched every time I walked in the door and then sent me back out again with increasingly severe assurances that the pain was "unwarranted" and probably all in my head.

After alienating every doctor in town with my complaints, I finally gave up and decided to 'suffer in silence' until one hot summer day almost twenty-four months after the birth, I suddenly fell, screaming with pain, on my living room floor in front of my terrified two year old. I literally had to crawl to the phone to call my husband. When he carried me, screeching, into my OB's office, the doctor clicked his tongue disapprovingly. "Now it can't be that bad, dear, we just checked you out a few months ago", he cajoled.

He gave me Codeine and sent me home – 48 hours later I was in the operating room having emergency surgery for multiple ruptured ovarian tumors.

A couple of days after the procedure, my doctor sauntered into my hospital room with a conciliatory grin on his face. "Gee", he drawled apologetically, "We had no idea anything like this was going to happen. Your ovary looked horrible – engorged to the size of a grapefruit. No wonder you were hurting. Sorry you had to go so long without help but, you know, the tests just never turned up anything. And oh, by the way, the pathologist found a little endometriosis in your right ovary."

Endometriosis is an incurable women's disease in which uterine tissue for some unknown reason detaches itself from the uterus, moves to other locations in the body, and attaches itself to other organs or body tissue. This misplaced uterine tissue spontaneously bleeds in response to hormonal changes, causing internal bleeding, scarring and often excruciating pain that can destroy the woman's ability to live and function normally. This disease is not uncommon among women, but it is incurable, at least by conventional medical standards.

My "little" endometriosis turned into the monster that ate Tokyo – three months after my doctor had "successfully" operated, I was sitting in the ultrasound room at the hospital again, watching as several new endometrial tumors appeared on the monitor screen, accompanied by the usual excruciating pelvic pain, internal bleeding, constipation, hemorrhagic cystitis and acute exhaustion.

After the ultrasound, I decided to contact a doctor who was recommended to me as an expert on endometriosis. He told me that he felt that my health problems had originally stemmed from undiagnosed severe endometriosis and an underactive thyroid which had probably been present since adolescence. He recommended an immediate hysterectomy, which I underwent. The day after the operation, the doctor visited me and compassionately whispered that I would "never have a problem with endometriosis again". But he was wrong.

Twenty months later, I had more tumors and another operation. Three months after that, the pain, tumors and internal bleeding reappeared again and I was scheduled for what would by now have been my sixth surgical procedure in five years, which I refused to undergo.

Desperate and seriously debilitated, I flew to Mexico where I spent $15,000 on an intensive course of intravenous mega-vitamin and live-cell therapy at one of the alternative cancer clinics which had offered some hope for my case. For weeks, doctors poured nutrients and natural medicines into my veins and mouth. I watched as many of the cancer patients around me seemed to get better and better with the treatments. And I did too – for about two months.

I spent my fortieth birthday hopelessly sick and in bed which was where I stayed that entire year. The drugs, operations and Mexican treatments had completely failed, and my usual herbs and homeopathic remedies, although they gave temporary relief, seemed almost useless against the disease. And by now, even though I had health insurance, my husband and I had spent over $100,000 of our own money, and still, I couldn't even get out of bed.

I had one last surgery which removed another large bleeding tumor. When I got home from the hospital, I weighed 89 pounds and developed a post-surgical infection which required several courses of antibiotics. After taking the antibiotics, I developed an extremely severe case of candida (yeast infection). My hands and arms became covered with a horribly itchy fungal infection that nothing could relieve or cure, and I remained generally exhausted, bedridden, and in intense pain.

Because of the surgeries, I was also experiencing early and severe menopausal symptoms – hot-flashes, mood swings, water retention and depression. But because endometriosis is exacerbated by estrogen, my doctor recommended that I refrain from taking estrogen supplements which she said would have relieved the severe and very unpleasant symptoms.

Several months after the surgery, the all-too-familiar endometrial symptoms returned. My doctor assured me that all was well, but when I asked for and received my surgical records from the hospital, I found that she had written that "all attempts to remove endometriosis will be done, but complete surgical care can rarely be guaranteed; the patient may require further therapy for endometriosis, medically or surgically." For my exhausted and bewildered husband and myself, this prognosis seemed like an insurmountable and final defeat.

I had one more heart to heart talk with a gynecologist who told me, "given the severity of your case, the reality is that you could be facing a lifetime of corrective surgery". Given the state of my health at the time, I couldn't envision that 'lifetime' meant anything more for me than a few additional years of mind-numbing pain and misery before my body finally gave out.

After nearly a lifetime of illness, these last episodes in my late thirties and early forties seemed like the final blow, and in all honesty I felt that there was no way out and no hope in sight. No matter how many times I'd been assured by my doctors that drugs and surgery would cure the endometriosis and my other disorders and make it possible for me to live a normal life, the doctors had been proven wrong.

A few weeks later, when I heard that one of my friends from the cancer clinic had died in his sleep, I felt sad for his family, but happy for him, because he was finally free of his pain and suffering. In many ways, I felt that he was the lucky one and I almost wished that the same thing would happen to me; it seemed that death would have been a blessing, especially so that my family could be freed from the seemingly never-ending burden of my illness and be able to get on with their lives.

Sitting alone and discouraged one morning, I glanced up dismally from a book I was reading when my husband came in the room. "I've got something else we can try, honey," he chirped enthusiastically, and proceeded to describe his conversation with a woman who had cured herself of a serious and reportedly incurable kidney disorder by using an unusual therapy. "Whaaat", I responded, after he told me what the therapy was – "I don't think so", I said, and went back to reading my book.

But after several more days and many more horrible episodes of pain and drugs, my husband handed me a small book and said, "You've got to try this". I picked up the book and began to read.

The small, unpretentious-looking book was full of fascinating stories about people who had been cured of even the worst diseases with a seemingly strange and little-known natural therapy. The therapy seemed incredibly effective, yet I still felt reluctant to try it. But as I read further on in the book, the stories were so compelling and the therapy was so simple that suddenly, it didn't seem strange or preposterous to me anymore. And at this point in my now nearly futile existence, I knew I had absolutely nothing to lose by trying it – so I did.

From the first day I began the therapy, to my immense surprise I got almost instantaneous relief from my incurable constipation and fluid retention. Within a week, my severe abdominal and pelvic pain was unbelievably gone.

The chronic cystitis and yeast infections (internal and external) soon disappeared and food allergies, exhaustion, and digestive problems all began to heal.

After a few more months of the therapy, I noticed that amazingly, my colds, flu, sore throats and viral symptoms, all of which had resurfaced and become chronic after the surgeries, now rarely made an appearance. My hair which had fallen out in handfuls after my fifth surgery became thick and lustrous, my weight normalized, and my energy and strength increased so markedly that I was even able to work again.

Last summer, I hiked four miles into the Grand Canyon. For the first time in many years I can swim and even comfortably ride horseback or on my mountain bike for hours at a time – all formerly unimaginable activities. Much to my own and my family's amazement, I am back at work and after 30 years of almost non-stop illness, I have a rich, full life again – and all because of an unbelievably simple and effective natural medicine that almost none of us even knows exists.

This natural therapy became, for me, a priceless gift of health, as it has for many others. It gave the fastest, most dramatic results of any natural or man-made medical treatment I have ever tried and was truly the miraculous happy ending to my long story of illness and failed medical treatments. By using this simple, natural medicine, along with other natural healing approaches such as homeopathy, herbs, good nutrition and rest, I have been able to remain consistently disease-free and I feel better and stronger than I have ever felt in my life since that fateful day in July so many years ago.

And even though this natural medicine seemed so peculiar to me at first, I later discovered, to my surprise, that medical researchers have been intensively studying and using this medicinal substance for decades.

As a matter of fact, unknown to the vast majority of the public, this incredibly simple and wonderful natural treatment is a well-proven medical therapy that has been used extensively and successfully throughout the twentieth century by doctors and researchers from many different branches of medicine all over the world and has been shown to be amazingly effective in treating a huge variety of illnesses.

It's time that all of us should know about this therapy and about the medical research findings on this truly remarkable natural medicine, which is why I have written this book.

Up until this point, whenever anyone wrote or talked about using this substance for healing, they've been told that it's just an unproven folk remedy or 'old wives tale'.

But as you'll discover in the following pages, this is completely untrue. The truth is that doctors and medical researchers for years have scientifically proven the tremendous effectiveness of this natural medicine – they just haven't told us about it, for reasons which we'll discuss later on in the book.

This simple, natural method may seem less glamorous than commercial drugs and space-age surgical techniques because it's not glorified by the press or hyped by sophisticated, sugar-coated advertising themes. But when all the man-made medicines in the world can't help, people like myself have been eternally grateful to find that nature has provided this safe, painless solution to even seemingly incurable illnesses.

In this age of hi-tech drugs, plastic body parts and mechanized medicine, I sincerely hope that all of us can become more open and accepting of this natural way of healing the body, and that the information provided in this book will help all of us to learn more about, (what I can unreservedly say), is the best natural remedy to disease and illness in existence.

CHAPTER TWO

WHAT MODERN SCIENCE KNOWS ABOUT A MIRACLE MEDICINE
(AND ISN'T TELLING)

Although the knowledge and research findings on this extraordinary natural medicine have largely remained in the files of medical researchers in our century, there are people who have inadvertently discovered the incredible healing power of this substance and have used it to heal themselves:

"I was officially diagnosed with Adenocarcinoma (cancer) of the chest with possible infiltration of the left lung two years ago. Soon after I was diagnosed, I was hospitalized because my lung had filled with fluid and collapsed. I was in a desperate struggle to stop the production of the fluid, in addition to which I was terribly constipated and uncomfortable.

Then I came across information on this particular natural therapy. As soon as I had ingested the [fluid] it was miraculous. My bowels immediately began to move again. The relief was incredible and the fluid production in my lung also subsequently soon died down to the doctors' amazement. They had no recourse but to remove my chest tube. They wanted me to consider chemotherapy, radiation or surgery but I refused and signed myself out of the hospital.

Needless to say I am still here after two years even though my parents were informed I had only four months to live after the diagnosis. I had used a number of holistic approaches (colonics, herbs, etc.) but to be perfectly honest I know it was the internal and external use of [this fluid] which has saved my life."

— **Mr. R.,**
   New York

"I was diagnosed as having rheumatoid arthritis at the age of twenty-eight. The pain and swelling in the joints of my hands was unbeliev-

able. I also suffered from migraine headaches since I was eight years old and it was very common for me to take a bottle of Excedrin with me everywhere I went. I never left my house without that bottle. I had also developed a severe weight problem over the years and had gotten up to almost 200 pounds.

Finally, I met someone who told me about this natural miracle therapy, but the best miracle of all is me. I started taking [this fluid] and four and a half months later I weighed 130 pounds. I lost 68 pounds! My arthritis is gone, my headaches are gone and I feel like I'm 20 years old.

— Mrs B.
Florida

"I laughed when I first heard about this therapy and didn't take it seriously. My main concern at the time was about my full-blown case of AIDS that had just been diagnosed and the Kaposi's sarcoma lesion (cancer) in my mouth that was supposed to spread throughout my body. But I decided to try the therapy topically on my vicious case of */ringworm and not only did the ringworm condition totally disappear after a few weeks, but the dry, cracked and painful skin all around my toes and foot had totally changed. New skin had grown in and was as soft as a baby's. It had a beautiful new color and just did not appear to be my own skin!

I then tried the therapy internally each day and over the next 7 months the Kaposi's lesions became increasingly smaller until they disappeared totally! The mouth ulcers and genital herpes that used to plague me have not returned even once. I have NEVER felt better in my life."

— Mr. Q.
New York

But it's not only people like these who have used this remarkable substance for healing. Medical scientists and doctors in the U.S. and all over the world have proven that this incredible body fluid and its components can actually destroy disease-causing viruses, bacteria and cancerous tumors, dissolve dangerous blood clots that cause heart attacks, heal ulcers, obesity, asthma, hay fever, allergies, colds, flu and digestive complaints as well as a host of other abnormalities and diseases.

This simple natural fluid contains one of the best and safest diuretic agents ever discovered. This agent has been proven to heal serious wounds and burns without scarring and is one of the most extraordinary natural skin moisturizers available.

After nearly 100 years of modern study, medical researchers, in reference to this fluid and its components, report these findings:

In clinical studies using an extract of this fluid on cancer patients, most patients in the study showed remarkable improvement after only one week of treatment and continued treatment produced a reduction in tumor size and normalization of biochemical tests with-out toxic or dangerous side effects.

— Dr. S. Burzynski
Physiology, Chemistry & Physics, 1977

It surprisingly and easily kills viruses. In strong concentration, it not only weakens viruses such as polio and rabies, but actually destroys them.

— Proceedings of the Society of Experimental Biology, 1936

Natural antibodies to the HIV virus appear in this fluid in patients diagnosed with AIDS.

— New York University Medical Center, 1988

Sufficiently concentrated, it will kill gonorrhea bacteria.

— Dr. Robert C. Noble
Division of Infectious Disease
University of Kentucky College of Medicine, 1987

It is capable of controlling a wide range of food, environmental and chemical allergies.

— Dr. C.M.W. Wilson
Department of Geriatric Medicine
Law Hospital, Scotland, 1983

It is capable of killing or stopping the growth of the bacteria that causes tuberculosis.

— The American Review of Tuberculosis, 1954

This agent is one of the safest and most useful diuretics known. Its use is indicated in the treatment of excess pressure on the brain and eyes, inoperable brain tumors, skull fractures, and cerebral contusions.

Further trials of this substance are warranted in the treatment of chronic glaucoma, hydrocephalus, delirium tremens, premenstrual edema, meningitis and epilepsy.

— **Symposium on Surgery
of the Head and Neck
Urea – New Use Of An Old Agent, 1957**

This substance acts as an excellent and safe natural vaccine and has been shown to cure a wide variety of disorders including chronic and acute hepatitis, whooping-cough, asthma, hayfever, hives, migraine and intestinal disfunctions. The method is so simple it can be used without any difficulties.
— **Dr. J. Plesch
Medical Press, London, 1947**

It was found that many physical illnesses were relieved, such as multiple sclerosis, colitis, hypertension, lupus, rheumatoid arthritis, hepatitis, hyperactivity, pancreatic insufficiency, psoriasis and eczema, diabetes, herpes zoster, and mononucleosis.

— **Dr. N. Dunne
Medical Advisor to the
Irish Allergy Treatment and Research Association
Oxford Medical Symposium, 1981**

Certain fractions of this substance have an inhibitory action on the growth of malignant tumors in mice...while smaller doses inhibit growth, bigger ones make the tumors regress.

— **Science Magazine, 1963**

More scientific papers have probably been published on this substance than on any other organic compound.

— **Journal of the American Medical Association
July 3, 1954**

So what is this mystery miracle medicine and why don't any of us know anything about it? If the body really does produce such an amazing substance, and doctors and scientists have used it to heal people, where are the news reports, the accolades, the commercials, the media hype?

You want to know the answer? Then prepare yourself by first opening your mind. Let go of your initial disbelief and preconceptions and get ready for the best-kept secret in medical history.

This extraordinary miracle medicine that numerous doctors, researchers and hundreds of people have used for healing is human urine.

Surprised? Now before you scream "I don't believe it" and slam the book shut, consider this: Whether you know it or not, you've already re-used and reingested your urine – large amounts of it for a long period of time, and it's one of the reasons you're alive today.

As medical researchers have discovered:

> *"Urine is the main component of the amniotic fluid that bathes the human fetus.*
>
> *Normally, the baby 'breathes' this urine-filled amniotic fluid into its lungs. If the urinary tract is blocked, the fetus does not produce the fluid, and without it, the lungs do not develop."*

> **— New York Times Medical Section,
>   August 16, 1988**

This is a fact that probably none of you without a medical background know –but the reality is, that urine is absolutely vital to your body's functioning and the internal and external applications of urine have proven medical ramifications far beyond anything that we, the general public can imagine.

It doesn't matter how violent your reaction or how strong your disbelief may be, by the time you finish reading this book you will be utterly convinced and astounded by what the medical community hasn't told us about this incredible, but almost completely publicly unrecognized natural medicine.

What amazes people most when they first hear about the medical use of urine is that they've never heard of it. To the vast majority of mankind, urine is nothing more than a somewhat repugnant "waste" that the body has to excrete in order to function.

But as you'll discover, urine is not a waste product of the body, but rather, an extraordinarily valuable physiological substance that has been shown throughout the history of medical science right up until today to have profound medical uses that most of us know absolutely nothing about.

One of the first things we need to clear up is the common perception of urine – urine is *not* what you think it is. As a matter of fact, you probably have no idea what urine is or how your body makes it.

In reality, urine is not, as most of us believe, the excess water from food and liquids that goes through the intestines and is ejected from the body. I know that we generally think of urine in just this way – you eat and drink, the intestines "wring" out the good stuff in the food, and the urine is the left-over, dirty waste water that your body doesn't want, so it should never, ever be reintroduced back into the body in any form – right? Wrong.

No matter how popular a conception this commonly shared scenario may be, it just isn't true. Urine is *not* made in your intestines. Urine is made in and by your kidneys. So what does this mean and why should it change the way you feel about urine?

In layman's language, this is how and why urine is made in the body: When you eat, the food you ingest is eventually broken down in the stomach and intestines into extremely small molecules. These molecules are absorbed into tiny tubules in the intestinal wall and then pass through these tubes into the bloodstream.

The blood circulates throughout your body carrying these food molecules and other nutrients, along with critical immune defense and regulating elements such as red and white blood cells, antibodies, plasma, microscopic proteins, hormones, enzymes, etc., which are all manufactured at different locations in the body. The blood continually distributes its load of life-sustaining elements throughout the body, nourishing every cell and protecting the body from disease.

As it flows through the body, this nutrient-filled blood passes through the liver where toxins are removed and later excreted from the body in the form of solid waste. Eventually, this purified, "cleaned" blood makes its way to the kidneys.

When the blood enters the kidneys it is filtered through an immensely complex and intricate system of minute tubules called nephron through which the blood is literally "squeezed" at high pressure. This filtering process removes excess amounts of water, salts and other elements in the blood that your body does not need at the time.

These excess elements are collected within the kidney in the form of a purified, sterile, watery solution called urine. Many of the constituents of this filtered watery solution, or urine, are then reabsorbed by the nephron and delivered back into the bloodstream. The remainder of the urine passes out of the kidneys into the bladder and is then excreted from the body.

So, you say, the body's gotten rid of this stuff for a reason – so why would we want to use it again? And here's the catch: **The function of the kidneys is to keep the various elements in your blood balanced. The kidneys do not filter out important elements in the blood because those elements in themselves are toxic or poisonous or bad for the body, but simply because the body did not need that particular concentration of that element at the time it was excreted.**

And medical researchers have discovered that many of the elements of the blood that are found in urine have enormous medicinal value, and when they are reintroduced into the body, they boost the body's immune defenses and stimulate healing in a way that nothing else does.

As medical research has revealed:

> *"One of the most important functions of the kidney is to excrete material and substances for which the body has no immediate need..."*

— Urinalysis in Clinical and Laboratory Practice

For instance, the kidneys filter out water and sodium from the blood into the urine. Are water and sodium toxic? Of course not, they're both vital life-sustaining elements without which your body cannot function. But both elements could be lethal if there were too much water or sodium in your blood.

Now what about potassium, calcium, and magnesium – these are familiar nutrients that we ingest in our food and vitamin pills everyday – but they're also in your urine. These nutritional elements are extremely valuable substances to the body, certainly not toxic, and yet the kidney excretes these elements into the urine – why? Because it's taking out the excess amount of the potassium, calcium, etc. that is not needed by your body at the time that they are filtered out. Actually, it is this regulating process of the kidneys and the excretion of urine that allows us to eat and drink more than our bodies need at any one time.

"The principal function of the kidney is not excretion, but regulation ... The kidney obviously conserves what we need, but even more, permits us the freedom of excess. That is, it allows us to take in more than we need of many necessities – water and salt for example – and excretes exactly what is not required."

— **Dr. S. Cameron**
   Prof. of Renal Medicine
   Guy's Hospital, London

But this isn't the end of the story. Scientists have discovered that urine, because it is actually extracted from our blood, contains small amounts of almost all of the life-sustaining nutrients, proteins, hormones, antibodies and immunizing agents that our blood contains:

"Urine can be regarded as one of the most complex of all body fluids. It contains practically all of the constituents found in the blood."

— **Urinalysis in Clinical and Laboratory Practice**

Many medical researchers, unlike most of us, know that far from being a dirty body waste, fresh, normal urine is actually sterile and is an extraordinary combination of some of the most vital and medically important substances known to man. Now this fact may be unknown to the vast majority of the public today, but, as you'll discover in this book, it is nothing new to modern medicine.

To us, the public, urine seems like an undesirable waste product of the body, but to the medical research community and the drug industry, it's been considered to be liquid gold. Don't believe it? Read this:

HIPPOCRATES MAGAZINE
May/June 1988

NOW URINE BUSINESS

Utica, Mich. – *Realizing it is flushing potential profits down the drain, an enterprising young company has come up with a way to trap* *medically powerful proteins from urine. Enzymes of America has designed a special filter that collects important urine proteins and these filters have been installed in all of the men's urinals in the 10,000 portable outhouses owned by the Porta-John company, a subsidiary of Enzymes of America.*

Urine is known to contain minute amounts of proteins made by the body, including medically important ones such as growth hormone and insulin. There is a $500-million-a year market for these kinds of urine ingredients.

This summer, Enzymes of America plans to market its first major urine product called urokinase, an enzyme that dissolves blood clots and is used to treat victims of heart attacks. The company has contracts to supply the urine enzyme to Sandoz, Merrell Dow and other major pharmaceutical companies. Ironically, this enterprise evolved from Porta-John's attempt to get rid of urine proteins – a major source of odor in portable toilets.

When the president of Porta-John began consulting with scientists about a urine filtration system, one told him he was sitting on a gold mine.

The idea of recycling urine is not new, however. "We thought about this," says Phillip Whitcome of Amgen, a Los Angeles biotechnology firm, "but realized we'd need thousands and thousands of liters of urine."

Porta-John and Enzymes of America solved that problem. The 14 million gallons flowing annually into Porta-John's privies contain about four and a half pounds of urokinase alone. That's enough to unclog 260,000 coronary arteries.

— Hippocrates Magazine

But urokinase isn't the only drug derived from urine that, unknown to us, has been a financial boon to the pharmaceutical industry.

In August of 1993, Forbes magazine printed an article about Fabio Bertarelli who owns the world's largest fertility-drug producing company called the Ares-Serono Group based in Geneva, whose most important product is the drug Pergonal which increases the chances of conception.

Guess what Pergonal is made from.

"To make Pergonal, Ares-Serono collects urine samples from 110,000 postmenopausal women volunteers in Italy, Spain, Brazil and Argentina. From 26 collection centers the urine is sent to Rome, where Ares-Serono technicians then isolate the ovulation-enhancing hormone."

— Forbes

Ares-Serono earned a reported $855 million in sales in 1992, and people pay up to $1,400 per month for this urine extract.

Obviously, most of us are operating under a gross misconception when we wrinkle our nose at the thought of using urine in medicine.

Urea, the principal organic solid in urine, has long been considered to be a "waste product" of the body – it's even been considered to be dangerous or poisonous, but this too is completely untrue.

Urea function

Like any other substance in the body, too much urea can be harmful, but urea in and of itself is enormously valuable and indispensable to body functioning. Not only does urea provide invaluable nitrogen to the body, but research has shown that urea actually aids in the synthesis of protein, or in other words, it helps our bodies use protein more efficiently. Urea has also been proven to be an extraordinary antibacterial and anti-viral agent, and is one of the best natural diuretics ever discovered.

Urea was discovered and isolated as long ago as 1773 and is currently marketed in a variety of different drug forms.

Another urine-related product ingredient is carbamide. Carbamide is the chemical name for synthesized urea. Where do you find carbamide? – in places you'd never thought of such as in products like Murine Ear Drops and Murine Ear Wax Removal System, which contain carbamide peroxide, a combination of synthetic urea and hydrogen peroxide.

Medical researchers have also proven that urea is *one of the best and only medically proven effective skin moisturizers in the world.*

These are a few more examples of commercial medical applications of urine and urea in use today:

Ureaphil: diuretic made from urea

Urofollitropin: urine-extract fertility drug

PureaSkin: urea cream for skin problems

Amino-Cerv: urea cream used for cervical treatments

Premarin: urine-extract estrogen supplement

Panafil: urea/papain ointment for skin ulcers, burns and infected wounds

In many years of laboratory studies researchers discovered that, unlike just about all other types of oil-based moisturizers that simply sit on the top layers of the skin and do nothing to improve water retention within skin cells (which gives skin its elasticity and wrinkle-free appearance), urea actually increases the water-binding capacity of the skin by opening skin layers for hydrogen bonding, which then attracts moisture to dry skin cells.

This is a remarkable fact considering that women spend *billions* of dollars a year on outrageously expensive skin moisturizers whose ingredients, even in tightly controlled double-blind comparison tests *(see Chapter 4),* don't even come close to hydrating dry skin as well as simple, inexpensive urea.

So as surprising as it seems, urine and urea do have an amazing and voluminous history in both traditional and modern medicine.

An article in the *New York State Journal of Medicine* in 1980 by Dr. John R. Herman, Clinical Professor of Urology at Albert Einstein College of Medicine in New York City, points out the general misconceptions regarding urine and its medical use:

> *"Autouropathy (urine therapy) did flourish in many parts of the world and it continues to flourish today...there is, unknown to most of us, a wide usage of uropathy and a great volume of knowledge available showing the multitudinous advantages of this modality ...*
>
> *Urine is only a derivative of the blood...If the blood should not be considered 'unclean', then the urine also should not be so considered. Normally excreted, urine is a fluid of tremendous variations of composition ...*
>
> *... Actually, the listed constituents of human urine can be carefully checked and no items not found in human diet are found in it. Percentages differ, of course, but urinary constituents are valuable to human metabolism ... "*

Look up urea in a medical dictionary. In *Mosby's Medical and Nursing Dictionary* urea is defined, not as a useless body waste, but as a systemic diuretic and topical skin treatment. It's also prescribed to reduce excess fluid pressure on the brain and eyes.

Uric acid, another ingredient of urine, is normally thought of as an undesirable waste product of the body that causes gout. But even uric acid has recently been found to have tremendous health-promoting and medical implications. Medical researchers at the University of California at Berkeley reported in 1982 that they have discovered that:

Uric acid could be a defense against cancer and aging.

It also destroys body-damaging chemicals called free radicals that are present in food, water and air and are considered to be a cause of cancer and breakdowns in immune function.

Uric acid could be one of the things that enable human beings to live so much longer than other mammals.

— Omni Magazine, Oct. 1982

Urine is a critically important body fluid that has fascinated medical science throughout the centuries. Medical scientists study urine with tremendous intensity because, unlike the public, they know that it contains innumerable vital body nutrients and thousands of natural elements that control and regulate every function of the body.

The research book on urine published in 1975, *Urinalysis in Clinical Laboratory Practice,* stated that:

"The magnitude of the attention which urine receives is attested to by a recent study which dealt with only the low-molecular weight constituents of human urine.

This publication revealed that more than 1,000 technical and scientific papers, related only to low molecular weight substances in urine, appeared in the medical and scientific literature in one (1) single year...

It is now recognized that the urine contains thousands of compounds, and as new, more sensitive analytical tools evolve, it is quite certain that new constituents of urine will be recognized."

So, whether we know it or not, urine does have an extremely important and undisputed place in medicine – and not just as a diagnostic tool or as an ingredient of various synthetic drugs.

As the research studies presented in Chapter Four illustrate, natural urine and simple urea have been used consistently and extensively by medical researchers and scientists over the entire course of the twentieth century and have been proven to be profoundly effective and comprehensive therapeutic medicines that even in their natural or basic forms can produce outstanding and amazing healing results.

Your first reaction once you've read the convincing research demonstrating urine's often startling medical uses may be a willingness to use it as long as it's altered enough to make it unrecognizable. Many people might consider a synthetic or chemically altered form of urine, such as urokinase, the blood clot dissolver, as preferable to using it as a natural medicine.

But as we'll discuss throughout the book, there are many reasons for using urine in its natural form, rather than as a synthetic drug or extract, not the least of which is the fact that there is no synthetic equivalent for individual urine and never will be, owing to the tremendous complexity and uniqueness of each person's urine constituents.

Just as nature produces no two people who are exactly the same, there are also no two urine samples in the world that contain exactly the same components. Your own urine contains elements that are specific to your body alone which are medicinally valuable ingredients tailor-made to your own health disorders.

How can that be? Because your urine contains hundreds of elements that are manufactured by your body to deal with your personal, specific health conditions. Your body is constantly producing a huge variety of antibodies, hormones, enzymes and other natural chemicals to regulate and control your body's functions and to combat diseases that you may or may not know you have.

Modern research and clinical studies have proven that the thousands of critical body chemicals and nutrients that end up in your individual urine reflect your individual body functions, and when reutilized, act as natural vaccines, antibacterial, antiviral, anti-cancer agents, hormone balancers, allergy relievers, etc., (talk about the perfect preventive care treatment!).

Many doctors have discovered and shown that it's extremely important to use our own natural urine in healing because extracts or synthetic drug forms of urine don't contain all of these individualized elements that address our personal, individual health needs.

like formula vs. breastmilk!

Another reason that many doctors have emphasized the use of the natural form of urine is that it does not produce side effects, whereas synthetic drugs and therapies all produce side effects, many of which are extremely dangerous.

29

As an example, the urine-extract drug called urokinase, which is used to dissolve dangerous blood clots, can cause serious abnormal bleeding as a side effect; but natural urine itself (which contains measurable amounts of urokinase) has been used medicinally even in extremely large quantities without causing side effects.

If you're not familiar with just how pervasive and extreme the risk of chemical drug-taking is, go to the library and look up a copy of The Physician's Desk Reference. This is the doctor's guide to every prescription and over-the-counter drug on the market, and every one of them is accompanied by a long list of ominous and frightening potential side effects.

On the other hand, in almost 100 years of laboratory and clinical studies on the use of the use of natural urine and simple urea in medicine, extraordinary results have been obtained, but NO toxic or dangerous side effects to the user have ever been observed or reported by either researchers or patients using the therapy.

As we've learned, urea, which is the principal solid ingredient of urine, has been synthesized and medically used with excellent results and with no side effects. But again, as you'll read in the next chapter, research has shown that whole urine can cure many disorders that urea cannot, because urine contains thousands of therapeutic agents, such as important natural antibodies, enzymes and regulating hormones that urea alone does not contain.

Urine therapy not only has dozens of successful research trials supporting it, but also thousands of success stories from people all over the world. As many people today have discovered, conventional medicine held no answers for either their chronic or acute illnesses and health disorders – but urine therapy did.

Learning More About One of the Biggest Secrets in Medical History

I realize that by now many of you are saying to yourselves, "All this information on the medical use of urine sounds fascinating, but can I really use this therapy at home? How would I get started, and how can I possibly get past my first fears and reluctance to try it for myself?"

GETTING STARTED

In reality, beginning the therapy is completely simple and painless. You're going to be starting the internal therapy with extremely small amounts. 1 to 2 drops is all that is needed as a first internal dose, and as medical research studies presented in Chapter 4 show, (see Dr. C.E. Lewis and Dr. N. Dunne), even a few drops can be therapeutically very effective. Also, if you prefer, you can make an extremely diluted form of urine called a homeopathic urine preparation, which gives excellent results and contains no taste or color. Chapter 6 contains complete and detailed instructions that will answer all your questions, including how to get started, how to prepare homeopathic urine, etc., and will make it easy for you to learn how to take advantage of this incomparable natural medicine in your everyday life.

HOW TO USE THE BOOK

There is so much information contained in this book, that it may all seem somewhat overwhelming at first; more than 50 research reports by doctors and medical scientists on the use of urine therapy are reviewed, and all are filled with extensive case studies, as well as the doctor's comments and observations on their studies.

If you have a specific disorder and feel that you don't want to read all of the studies in order to get to the one that applies to you, look up your condition in the Index listing which will tell you where the information on your disorder is located in the book. Also, make sure that you read the instructions in Chapter 6 before beginning the therapy.

The use of urine in medicine is such a huge and previously untouched consumer subject that reading, organizing and compiling the pertinent information has presented quite a challenge. So to make it more comprehensible, I've devoted each chapter to particular, specific issues related to the medical use of urine.

The first and second chapters have been a general introduction to the largely unknown medical uses of urine and its importance as a natural medicinal.

In Chapter 3, we'll discuss why medical practitioners and the general public know nothing about the medical applications of urine even though there are centuries of historical anecdotes and volumes of modern scientific reports advocating its value. We'll also discuss more about why the use of the natural form of urine is preferable to urine extracts.

Chapter 4 is an in-depth look at selected laboratory and clinical studies conducted by doctors and researchers on the medical applications and significance of urine therapy. These extensive research studies span a period of almost an entire century.

Chapter 5 presents the interesting history of the use of urine therapy around the world.

Chapter 6 contains directions for home use.

Chapter 7 presents personal testimonials on specific disorders and disease conditions.

In these days of anxiety and fear about health care, perhaps the most important thing for all of us to remember is that <u>knowledge is our greatest strength and our best health insurance.</u> The more we know about our bodies and how to use simple, safe remedies to correct diseases and chronic illnesses, the healthier and happier each one of us will be.

By the time you finish reading everything that people, doctors and scientists have to say about urine therapy, you will agree, without a doubt, that it's one of the best and most valuable medical secrets that any of us have ever discovered. The medicinal properties of urine are so comprehensive and so astounding, yet so easily accessible that it gives each one of us amazing personal power over our own health that we never even knew we possessed – the cost-free, natural healing power of our own perfect medicine.

WHY NOBODY KNOWS ANYTHING ABOUT THE MOST RESEARCHED NATURAL SUBSTANCE IN MEDICINE

One of the questions that I'm most asked about urine therapy is: "If it's so wonderful and there's so much scientific evidence supporting it, why don't my doctors and the public know about it and why isn't it more widely used?"

Historically, the medical use of urine was quite well known throughout the world. There are many reports that date back thousands of years, (see Chapter Five), which extol the virtues of urine both as a diagnostic tool and as a medicinal treatment for a wide variety of diseases, wounds and skin disorders.

And yet today, even after nearly 100 years of consistent and authoritative modern medical research showing urine or urea to be one of the simplest, cheapest, most effective medicinal substances in existence, the vast majority of us, including even our own doctors, still mistakenly believe that urine is nothing more than a body waste or a medical diagnostic tool.

About all that consumers today know about urine in medicine is that you hand a sample of it to the doctor's nurse when you go for an office visit so they can test it for whatever it is that they test it for. And it's pretty much the same for the doctors.

So how have we and our doctors, who are supposed to know about these things, completely missed thousands of years of historical references and almost a century's worth of definitive modern research discoveries on the medical use of urine?

To really understand why the extensive medical use of urine is largely unknown and unpublicized today, we have to look more closely at the background and the history of modern medicine.

Before the advent of modern medicines, there were few man-made drugs, and even fewer doctors to administer them –and, for most people, no money for to pay the doctors even when they were available. So people generally treated their illnesses with prayer and such common sense approaches as good food, rest and whatever substances they found in nature that were traditionally known to have medicinal qualities – things like simple herbs, plants, minerals, urine, etc.

This natural approach to healing had recognizable benefits and even well-known and historically respected doctors such as Hippocrates taught that the body's own natural defenses should be supported and emphasized in healing and that gentle, natural medical approaches should always be used first before resorting to stronger interventions.

But throughout the known history of man and medicine, there has always been a type of "tug of war" going on between those who felt that nature was the best healer, and others who were convinced that man could intellectually devise healing techniques that would put Mother Nature to shame.

One of the most potent arguments on the side of those who favored science over nature were the various historical plagues of infectious diseases such as smallpox, typhoid, dysentery and the dreaded bubonic or "black plague" that would intermittently strike and wipe out millions of people in record time. Traditional medical approaches seemed of little use against such plagues, and westerners in particular began to search science for methods of overcoming these diseases.

During the late nineteenth and early twentieth centuries, science did discover man-made synthetic drugs like penicillin that seemed to prevent these killer plagues and other dangerous illnesses, and the age of modern synthetic medicine began. By the time the second half of the twentieth century had rolled around, mankind's scientific advances in medicine had produced a wide variety of sophisticated drugs and technology that seemed to make traditional health approaches obsolete.

Apparently, mankind and technology had finally won the battle against nature. In some ways, it appeared that humanity had even overcome its dependence on God; as Robert Koch, who first discovered microbes commented, "In the nineteenth century, man lost his fear of God and gained a fear of microbes." And perhaps this is true, because, unlike our great-grandparents and other ancestors back to the beginning of time, most modern societies today depend much more on drugs and medical science than on God, or the medicines that nature provides for healing disease or correcting health disorders. This is largely because today's medical community has conditioned us to believe that medical science, drugs and surgery are all that are needed to keep humanity healthy, happy and disease-free.

Medical science, not God and prayer, is now offered as our hope for increased longevity and a type of immortality, as scientists experiment with such things as cryogenics (freezing the body so that it can be 'resurrected' by future scientists), and surgical organ transplants that seem as though they could possibly extend our physical lives indefinitely. When infertility occurs, we can now turn, not to nature, or spiritual, or even psychological understanding, which often seem to fail to give us what we want, but to the mechanical manipulations of medical science which allow us to simply 'detour' around frustrating and 'unfair' natural impediments.

In view of all of the apparent advances and advantages of twentieth century medical science, the simpler, traditional and more natural approaches to medicine like urine therapy have appeared to be useless and ineffective to us, and we were right to have abandoned them in favor of 'objective' scientific medicine – or so we thought.

The book, *The Betrayal of Health,* published in 1991 by Dr. Joseph Beasely, M.D., a medical doctor and former Harvard University administrator and dean of the School of Public Health at Tulane University, simply and eloquently tells the story of the development of modern medicine and its unfortunate, unforeseen consequences:

> *"From the earliest days of medical science there have been two distinct but complementary approaches to health – the pursuit of well-being (the naturalistic school) and the cure of disease (the allopathic school).*
>
> *Hippocrates combined both approaches in his practice and medical teachings – stressing that the physician must be skilled in Nature and understand the patient in relation to his or her food, drink, and occupation, as well as the effect each of these factors has on the others.*
>
> *Health was an equilibrium between the mind and body and the external world, disease a disruption of this natural harmony.*
>
> *Treatment involved creating the conditions in which the body could maintain and cure itself through its internal healing mechanisms. When disease did manifest itself, specific intervention would be applied, but natural cures such as dietary changes were preferred over drugs."*

But as Dr. Beasley points out, this balanced, natural approach to medicine did not survive the twentieth century avalanche of enthusiasm for sophisticated synthetic drugs and surgery that seemingly freed us from the scourges of infectious disease epidemics and other serious illnesses:

> *"The modern approach to illness and health developed over centuries of battles against a host of diseases. During most of those years, medicine was not particularly effective. Plagues and contagions wiped out entire populations as medical practitioners labored in vain to find a cure.*
>
> *These centuries of medical failure made the relatively recent century of medical success all the more impressive."*

As Dr. Beasley states, the medical community and the public became so sure that science could find a specific drug cure for every illness that everyone totally ignored the importance of factors like natural medicines, nutrition, environment and mental health in creating and maintaining good health:

> *"The discovery and destruction of the germs responsible for disease led doctors (and their patients) to place their faith in the scientific [medical] model that had so miraculously saved humanity from its most ancient enemies.*
>
> *But in the process of developing modern medical methods, medicine has abandoned (or forgotten) some of its most ancient and worthwhile traditions.*
>
> *The complex interactions of nutrition were neglected even as they were being discovered. And there has been even less interest in the interactive effects of environmental agents or of long-term behavioral patterns on health."*

The seemingly enormous healing power of new synthetic drugs appeared to make common sense natural approaches to medicine obsolete. Now that we had miracle antibiotics that could apparently cure everything and powerful pain relievers and new, fantastic surgical techniques, who needed outmoded, unsophisticated natural medical approaches like urine therapy or nutrition or homeopathy or herbs?

As the twentieth century progressed, people didn't treat themselves at home anymore with time-honored natural remedies. If you got sick, instead of treating yourself with more rest, better food and a simple traditional natural medicine, you went to the doctor or the drug store to buy whatever 'miracle' drug was popular at the time, or you had an operation.

In our century, drug companies, and the medical researchers they hired, took the job of making and experimenting with medicines away from doctors and the public and withdrew into their laboratories.

In scientific seclusion, far removed from the world of the doctor-patient relationship, researchers experimented with chemical compounds and isolated medically active ingredients in natural substances such as previously well-known herbs or urine, and then formulated drugs from these elements.

In the case of urine therapy, urine was used in its natural form or as simple urea in numerous clinical tests throughout our century, but these studies were never publicized, because, for the most part, the use of natural medicines had been discontinued in medical practice in favor of patented drugs and surgery.

With our new system of modern medicine, people no longer felt that it was necessary or important for them to know how their bodies worked or how to treat themselves with simple methods at home. Most consumers felt that the knowledge of the body and how to heal it was best left in the hands of scientists and trained doctors and surgeons who knew so much more than we did about how to manipulate and alter the body and defeat disease.

In this scenario, the use of urine therapy wasn't important to the public. No one talked about it or shared the information with their family and friends as they had in days gone by. And even though modern researchers were discovering amazing things about urine therapy, these discoveries were kept within the walls of academic research and were never or rarely shared with the public.

But were we right to abandon traditional and common sense approaches to healing? Should natural healing methods like urine therapy have a place in our lives or should we just continue to completely surrender our personal health-care needs and concerns to doctors and medical researchers? Are chemical drugs and surgery really the answer to all our health problems? As most of us are aware today – they're not.

No matter how many incredible discoveries medical science may have made during the twentieth century, millions of us are sick or even crippled by illness today. Our doctors don't know what to do. Our scientists continue to tell us that science, drugs and surgery will cure us, but they don't.

As *The Betrayal of Health* points out, our modern miracle medicine is not the miracle we thought it was:

> *"As the infectious diseases became less and less prevalent, and the chronic diseases advanced to the forefront of illness, cracks have begun to appear in the fortress of allopathic medicine. The methods that had produced the successes of Jenner, Pasteur, Koch, Fleming and Salk no longer seemed to be working. Further, flaws in, and abuses of, modern medical techniques have become all too apparent.*
>
> *The unqualified successes of earlier decades have come up against the failures of modern medicine.*
>
> *The epidemic of chronic illness in the United States, particularly arterial disease and cancer, is the stellar embarrassment of medicine and its high-technology weapons.*
>
> *These degenerative illnesses – far from being bull's eye illnesses – are complex dysfunctions of bodily systems that must be approached systematically.*
>
> *With them, the model of specific cause/specific medical intervention simply isn't working. What is worse, many interventions, from prescription drugs to expensive surgery, cause more harm than good when they are overused or abused by doctors and patients.*
>
> *Ironically, the wonder drugs of the last century may never have worked as well as we thought. Medical historians report that the dramatic improvements in morbidity and mortality rates in the past hundred years were not exclusively, nor even mainly, due to doctors' intervention.*
>
> *The great health improvements of the nineteenth century were not the result of medical interventions per se, but of basic improvements in nutritional and living conditions that coincided with (and often preceded) these interventions."*

So even though we believed that drugs and medical science alone were responsible for saving us from smallpox and typhoid and other terrible diseases, this was never true. The truth was that we got fewer infectious diseases in the twentieth century because we had better living conditions. For the first time in history, we had widespread modern sanitation, clean water and more and better food distribution than ever before. In the modern environment of civilized nations, infectious diseases disappeared because the breeding grounds for germs, such as open sewers, contaminated water supplies and malnourished bodies were largely eliminated.

But medical science undeservedly took and received the greatest credit and public acclaim for these tremendous health improvements. And the medical community today is still trying to convince us that no matter what goes wrong with our bodies, the solution will always be found within the realm of drugs and surgery.

It is true that drugs and surgery can be extremely effective for critical care, health emergencies, structural deformities or accident cases, but these aggressive therapies should never have developed into everyday medical approaches that we automatically resort to almost immediately for every imaginable illness we contract.

Western culture made a grave error when it eliminated all natural approaches to health in favor of drugs and surgery. Natural healing methods that gently stimulate and support the immune system without dangerous side effects have advantages that drugs and surgery can't offer. And it wasn't that traditional natural health therapies, such as urine therapy, hadn't worked in the past – it was simply that historically they weren't always applied within the context of good nutrition and sanitation and proper health practices because this knowledge wasn't available in the centuries preceding ours.

And as Beasely points out, it was extremely ironic that even though modern science has proven the importance and impact of such common sense factors as diet and relaxation on health, the medical community and consumers have almost completely ignored these findings.

For instance, if a typical consumer today is having trouble falling asleep, chances are the person will immediately resort to Nytol, or Sominex, or whatever sleeping pill he or she saw advertised and promoted by drug companies on TV, and never even consider or try simple natural solutions such as taking a walk or warm bath, or drinking a soothing cup of tea, or eliminating the late-night snack of pepperoni pizza that's upsetting the stomach and causing insomnia – even though there is clear scientific evidence, not to mention common sense, that indicates that relaxation and dietary changes can help promote good sleep.

This same contradiction is also true for urine therapy. Medical scientists have proven the medical efficacy of natural urine and urea over and over again, but the medical community and drug companies have completely ignored these research findings – unless of course, a patentable drug form of urine such as Pergonal or Urokinase, can be developed.

It's unfortunate that even as most people and practicing doctors forgot about the use of natural urine therapy, medical researchers were discovering incredible things about the medicinal value of urine.

During this century, researchers sat in their laboratories and watched as simple urea or whole urine completely destroyed rabies and polio viruses, tuberculosis, typhoid, gonorrhea, dysentery bacteria and cancer cells.

They found that urine contains a huge array of incredibly valuable and medically important elements and they injected and orally administered urine and urea to thousands of patients in clinical tests.

They watched as it saved the lives of cancer patients, cured and relieved asthma, eczema, whooping cough, migraines, diabetes, glaucoma, rheumatoid arthritis, and a host of other illnesses. But the general public was never told about such discoveries.

Doctors and consumers today are given access to urine-related drugs, but have no idea of the tremendous overall value and health benefits of the natural urine that the drug was derived from. And medical researchers see absolutely no reason why any of us should know about it. All we need to know, in their estimation, is that they've developed a drug for a disease and where or what it's derived from is of little or no importance.

So why are many people like myself now resurrecting and using natural urine therapy instead of using sophisticated 'wonder' drugs and surgery? The answer is simple – drugs and surgery didn't work, but urine therapy did.

Urine therapy is regaining attention today because as the twentieth century draws to a close, millions of people are becoming aware that the keys to good health do not lie in the laboratory or the operating room.

Many of us now realize that when we threw out our natural medical approaches and methods of self-care, we eliminated crucially important elements in healing that can't be replaced by drugs or surgery. Unlike naturally occurring medicines, chemical drugs are extremely concentrated synthetic substances. Yes, these abnormally high concentrations may seem to produce a "knock-out punch" to disease symptoms, but what good is it if the drug delivers the same knock-out punch to your health as a whole?

We may think we're winning the battle against disease, but we all know we're losing the war. The AIDS epidemic and the other modern health epidemics of cancer, heart disease, diabetes, chronic fatigue syndrome, debilitating allergies, auto-immune diseases, ulcers, etc. aren't being cured by modern medicine. And one of the biggest reasons for this failure is that these modern epidemics are immune deficiency diseases which cannot be treated by immune-suppressing therapies such as drugs and surgery.

In fact, every single drug or surgical technique that exists in some way weakens and impairs our immune system functions, so it's impossible for these methods to cure the immune-deficiency diseases that are now killing and
maiming us.

The health epidemics of today are the consequences of many environmental factors that strain and break down our bodies' natural immune defenses, so drugs and surgery which further weaken our immune systems do absolutely nothing to cure or help us. They seem to temporarily win the battle against the symptoms of illness, but in the end they lose the war because they suppress and destroy the very thing that makes and keeps us well – our own natural body defenses.

Natural urine therapy was abandoned and forgotten by the public in the twentieth century because we were so sure that drugs and surgery were the answers to all our health problems. But time has shown us our error.

As we watch the often terrible and fatal consequences of decades of complete reliance on immune-suppressing synthetic drugs and surgical techniques unfold, we worriedly search the pages of history to rediscover and relearn the lost arts of caring for ourselves with simple, safe, and healthful natural healing.

Urine therapy is a natural therapy that is not widely known today, but in reality, it is not a lost healing art. As the material in this book shows, urine therapy has been kept very much alive by modern medical science throughout the twentieth century, even though it has rarely been publicized.

In reality, urine therapy cannot even be accurately classed as a traditional folk-remedy today, because during the twentieth century it has been used almost exclusively by mainstream medical scientists and researchers and not by consumers themselves, but this is changing.

So, in conclusion, it is the "surgery and drugs are all we need" philosophy of the present conventional medical system that is one major reason why you and your doctors have never heard of urine therapy. But there is another big reason why so many know so little about the world's least expensive and most powerful and effective natural medicine – very simply stated – there's no money in urine therapy.

Medicine and Money

I think that most of us are under the impression that somewhere in the sequestered halls of academia, benevolent doctors and research scientists are altruistically slaving over their petri dishes and test tubes, feverishly searching for new medical methods and cures that will relieve and eradicate physical suffering and illness – and that as soon as they make these wondrous new discoveries they'll immediately release the results of their studies to a desperately expectant world of sick and suffering people.

But as true as we want this scenario to be, it isn't the reality. The reality is that medical researchers are not the ones who ultimately decide what medical treatments the public receives as a result of medical research studies.

The architects of today's medical system are not primarily medical researchers or doctors, but rather, the drug companies. Medical research requires funding and from the very beginning of the age of modern medicine, researchers have largely depended on pharmaceutical companies to supply those funds. So many times we hear what the companies, and not the researchers, want us to hear about research discoveries.

The great pharmaceutical advances of the early 1900's that gave us the first new vaccines, penicillin, antitoxins and the 'miraculous' sulfa drugs were financed in large part by big pharmaceutical companies like Bayer and I.G. Farben. Now, while the owners of these drug companies may have had some altruistic interests, the lifeblood of their companies was not medicine, but money.

Simple, inexpensive medicines like herbs, homeopathic remedies or urine therapy that have been shown to be just as effective, safer and much less expensive than chemical drug compounds may be better for the public but they're no good for drug company profits and are therefore not promoted and sold.

It's in the drug industry's best interest to ignore and invalidate medicines and traditional therapies that can't be patented and don't produce big profits. And in simple economic terms, this is how any business survives and prospers – by selling and promoting the products that make the most money. Pharmaceutical firms by their very nature must promote profit-making medicines to keep their companies alive.

The way our medical system works today, drug companies are the primary entities that fund research, and test and prepare medical treatments for government approval, and this is also true in many countries throughout the world.

And it's extremely expensive for a company to conduct research for a new method and get it through the approval process – to do this can cost as much as an estimated $150 million per treatment. So a pharmaceutical company has to promote the medical approaches that will assure big "pay offs" in order for the company to survive.

Unfortunately, medicines that keep drug companies alive and healthy, even if they're government approved, can often make people sick – or even kill them.

Drugs like DES and thalidomide may have been big profit makers but they later created horrible health disorders and hideous fetal deformities when used by trusting consumers. Metabolic synthetic steroids, once hailed as miracle muscle-builders and used freely, are now killing and maiming many of their users. Aspirin was considered to be the ultimate miracle fever and pain reducer until it was discovered that it causes the Reyes syndrome that can kill children and can also cause severe abdominal bleeding in adults.

The fact is that no matter how much research or how many amazing or successful clinical trials have been performed by researchers on safe, inexpensive medical approaches like urine therapy, if these therapies are not perceived as profitable by pharmaceutical companies, they will simply not be 'picked up' by the drug companies and presented for government approval, which means that the public will probably never hear about the research or receive the benefits of these substances, no matter how wonderful they are.

The U.S. Food and Drug Administration (FDA) does not generally research or test medical treatments itself – it depends on private companies to do that. And because of this fact, the FDA does not have first-hand knowledge of which treatments are effective and safe and which aren't; they rely on the company that has developed the treatment to tell them which treatments should be marketed to consumers.

As the book, *The Betrayal of Health* reveals:

> *"The drug industry is a business. In a regrettable Catch-22, the main sources of information for the regulation of the pharmaceutical industry are the companies themselves. The 'watchdog' of the drug industry, the Food and Drug Administration, sets testing standards and then evaluates the test results submitted by the companies.*
>
> *In determining whether a drug is 'safe', the FDA does not perform clinical trials of new drugs and only rarely runs toxicity tests.*
>
> *As a result, the FDA must make its decisions based on information provided by the very company that wants to market the drug. If the information provided is fraudulent, the FDA (and the public) is unlikely to find out about it until a significant problem occurs...*
>
> *Despite the conflict of interest inherent in such situations, drug companies continue to be the major funder of research on most common diseases and their potential treatment.*
>
> *And it is no surprise that the research focuses on finding new chemical methods of managing disease – or at least symptoms. Indeed, could one expect A.H. Robbins or SmithKline or Ciba-Geigy to fund research on therapies (such as nutrition) that cannot be patented and will not significantly increase their market share?"*

The results of this unfortunate mix of medicine and money are reflected by the lack of attention given to research findings on urine and urea therapy. For example, urea, has been shown to be a much safer, simpler, less expensive and more effective diuretic than the diuretic drug, Diamox (see Urea – New Use Of An Old Agent, next chapter). Yet, in The Physician's Desk Reference, Diamox is mentioned under the diuretic category, but urea isn't – unlike simple urea, Diamox is a patented compound drug, insuring that the company's profits from the drug will be maximized and protected.

Another example of how money and medicine don't mix is the conventional medical community's treatment of medicinal herbs. There are numerous research studies proving the effectiveness, safety and diverse medical applications of herbs, yet any conventional doctor you talk to will tell you that herbal medicine is ridiculously unscientific and ineffective.

Doctors tell you this, not because it's true, but because their medical training is completely centered around drug and surgery treatments promoted by the pharmaceutical industry.

In the book, *The Scientific Validation of Herbal Medicine,* the author, Daniel Mowrey, lists hundreds of scientific studies that not only validate the medicinal effectiveness of herbs, but in many cases, prove that the natural herb or herbal extract can be just as effective as its synthetic counterpart.

For instance, the herb Cinchona was originally used for treating malaria and has been clinically proven to be just as effective as the synthetic drug quinine – and the herb is safe and non-toxic.

But even though millions of pounds of Cinchona were imported for medical use into the U.S. before the development of synthetic quinine, drug companies today would never consider recommending or advertising Cinchona. Why? Because synthetic drugs, unlike herbs or other simple medicines, can be patented and sold for much more profit.

And unfortunately, if the drug companies do not present a natural therapy such as urine therapy to the FDA for approval because it's unprofitable for them, the therapy doesn't get approved for use. That means that neither you or your doctor will hear about it or use it.

Urea is approved by the FDA and is used, as you've read, in several different commercial forms. But urea itself is extremely inexpensive and non-patentable so the truly important and often astounding medical breakthroughs using simple urea in research studies have never been given proper recognition, even though the researchers themselves have often stressed its importance and made repeated but unsuccessful attempts to bring the information to the attention of the medical community.

Consumers, and especially doctors, over the last 50 years have been thoroughly and completely indoctrinated with the "a drug a day keeps disease away" promotion of the drug companies, and have neglected the simpler, safer methods like natural urine or urea therapy. But how do we know that our doctors are right and that the drug companies are telling the truth when they say that the drugs we're taking are safe and effective and will heal the health disorders that we're taking them for?

Chemical Drugs – How Safe and Effective Are They?

Many people are afraid to try urine therapy because it's not recommended by conventional doctors. And our doctors, if we ask them, will tell us that they've never heard of it and if they have, they don't recommend it because it's never been proven safe or effective, whereas the drugs they prescribe are scientifically proven safe and effective and therefore have passed FDA approval testing. Drug companies and researchers tell us the same things about their drugs.

And like the uninformed health-care consumers that so many of us are, we believe them. But this information is, simply speaking, a big, fat lie.

The statement that medical therapies like urine therapy or herbal medicines are dangerous, unproven or "quackery", and that only FDA approved drugs and therapies are safe and effective is a blatant falsehood.

As you'll see after reading the research studies in the next chapter, not only does urine therapy have enormous scientific proof and validity on its side, but, unlike drugs and surgery, *not one person has ever suffered adverse side effects or died while using urine and urea medicinally in nearly 100 years of scientific scrutiny and use.*

On the other hand, *of the more than 300,000 over-the-counter medicines that are available to anyone at anytime off any drug store or grocery store shelf, only 1/3 of them have ever been demonstrated to be safe or effective and all are proven to have dangerous potential side effects and overdoses can even cause death.*

And don't take my word for it. Listen to what a large group of medical research scientists and doctors say about this issue in the book they wrote in 1983, entitled Over The Counter Pills That Don't Work. This book is a real eye opener, and will make you realize that just because a substance is FDA approved, available over the counter in the store, or doctor recommended, it has not necessarily been proven safe and effective:

> "...*Every day, on television, on the radio, in newspapers, in magazines, drug companies spend millions of your dollars to tell you about the wonders of their special and 'unique' over the counter drugs...*"

But fewer than 1/3 of these over the counter drug ingredients have been shown to be safe and effective for their intended uses.

In other words, many OTC [over-the- counter] drug products which you purchase contain one or more ingredients which do not meet the Federal drug law standards for safety, effectiveness, or both.

Of the more than 10 billion dollars Americans spend each year on OTC drugs, at least 3 or 4 billion dollars are wasted on grossly overpriced products or products with ingredients lacking evidence of safety or effectiveness.

Since all drug ingredients have risks, extra ingredients which aren't effective or which lack evidence of effectiveness subject you to extra risks without providing compensating benefits. So you are not only wasting your money when you buy products with such ingredients, but you are also risking your health and that of your family.

Starting 10 years ago, the U.S. Food and Drug Administration (FDA) established a large number of over the counter drug advisory panels – including physicians, pharmacists and other technically qualified people. They reviewed...the ingredients contained in approximately 300,000 brands of (OTC) drugs to determine if these ingredients were safe or effective...according to the FDA's Director of OTC Drug Evaluation, Dr. William Gilbertson, only 'about 1/3 of the ingredients reviewed by the panels have been shown to be safe and effective for their intended uses.'

FDA officials under pressure from the OTC drug companies have not implemented the findings of their panel."

The hundreds of drugs shown to be unproven for safety and effectiveness include well-known and widely used drugs like NyQuil, Alka-Seltzer, Bayer, Bufferin, Dristan, Anacin, Excedrin, Cope, 'doctor recommended' Preparation H and many more.

The same doctors and medical researchers who wrote this book on over-the-counter drugs, also wrote a consumer book on the dangers of prescription drugs entitled, *Pills That Don't Work:*

> *"You go to the doctor because you don't feel well. You are listened to (sometimes), examined, tested and then the doctor usually writes one or more prescriptions for you. You go to the drug store to have the prescriptions filled. You go home and start taking the pills. Now everything will be all right, right? Wrong.*
>
> ***Neither you nor, in some instances, even your doctor realizes that one out of every eight prescriptions filled...is for a drug not considered effective by the government's own standards.*** *Since all drugs involve risks, this lack of effectiveness means you are exposing yourself to dangers without gaining compensating benefits.*
>
> *In other words, balancing the benefits versus the risks, these drugs are not safe..."*

Health care consumers today are witnessing and experiencing firsthand the collapse of a medical system based on profit and saturated with the mistaken assumption that man-made drugs can be guaranteed to be safe and can completely usurp the healing power of nature and the use of safe natural healing methods.

Unfortunately, consumers in many cases are learning this error in medical thinking the hard way. A recent news-paper article on a new drug for the 'incurable' virus, hepatitis B, illustrates just how deadly this thinking can be:

Human Guinea Pig Says He's Lucky to Be Alive

Associated Press – Paul Melstrom of Phoenix warned the National Institutes of Health that the test drug he had taken was causing serious side effects. But no one listened.

Now, he lives with a painful nerve disorder, but still considers himself lucky. Five other people who tested the drug are dead.

Officials at the Institutes in Bethesda, Md., the premier federal medical research agency, acknowledge that the test went terribly wrong.

"Catastrophe" is how Dr. Jay H. Hoofnagle of the Institutes, who oversaw the original study, described it.

The federal Food and Drug Administration, which had given approval for the human trials is investigating what went wrong.

And this is not an isolated incident. As *The Betrayal of Health* points out, drug safety testing by drug companies is seriously flawed, because of the pharmaceutical industry's desire to continually pump out new, even if speculative, drug treatments:

"These speculative drug 'hand grenades' have done considerable damage over the course of pharmaceutical history. The best-known example was the tragedy of thalidomide, the tranquilizer that resulted in thousands of deformed children in Europe and Great Britain.

Yet the pharmaceutical industry continues to produce and market drugs that have the potential to cause a comparable tragedy..."

American consumers in particular are at risk from the side effects and consequences of medical drug abuse, because we take so many medications habitually:

The Wall Street Journal
Tuesday, January 11, 1994

"Americans as a society are over medicated, some experts say, because of a culture that no longer makes allowances for pain. Advertisements on television or in magazines, they say, have left the impression that there is a pill to make every pain or problem go away...

But consumers may nevertheless find themselves in the doctor's office either for complications arising from prolonged use of over-the-counter drugs themselves or for failing to recognize the [underlying] presence of a more serious illness."

Another problem with our reliance on synthetic drugs is that medical scientists try to prove that synthetic drugs are safe and effective by doing "conclusive" double-blind studies that are supposed to eliminate risk factors and show that a specific drug will work a certain way on everyone that has the disorder that the drug is supposed to treat.

But one important thing we have to remember in caring for ourselves is that t*here is no such thing as a generalized body or a specific cause for every illness.*

And in reality, there is no such thing as a completely conclusive double-blind drug study because no two people are exactly the same even if they happen to have the same disease. So the drug that works for one person might not work well at all for another person even though both have 'identical' disorders. As a result, no double-blind drug study is ever going to be completely objective or ultimately prove how a drug will affect everyone who takes it, which is another reason why drug fatalities and unforeseen side effects occur.

We think that we can blindly trust the FDA and our doctors, simply because they say we can – but blind faith can be deadly.

Health care in the U.S. is in crisis today, but the problem isn't too little money, it's too little attention being given to our bodies' real health needs, such as the critical need to support and enhance our bodies' own natural defenses against disease through traditional methods and com-mon sense approaches such as good nutrition, a balanced lifestyle, suf-ficient rest, and simple, safe, natural medicines.

I've asked doctors and medical practitioners many times about urine therapy and, if they've ever even heard of it, (99% of them haven't), they invariably tell me that, unlike the drugs they prescribe and recommend, it's not safe, it's an old wives tale, and it's never been proven effective.

But the truth is that urine therapy is proven and is safe, far more so than chemical drugs. And in view of the real facts about drugs and the drug industry it's frighteningly obvious that the real, substantiated risks are not those posed by correctly used proven natural healing approaches like urine therapy, but by routine, unnecessary surgeries and by dangerous prescription and over-the-counter chemical drugs that are marketed as freely as food, clothing and laundry soap.

What's Wrong With Urine Extracts?

After reading the medical research on urine people are always impressed, but they often ask if it wouldn't be easier and better to use it as an extract or drug. But in addition to the health problems and side effects that drugs create, there are other reasons why urine extracts and drugs can't replace natural urine therapy.

When it comes to personal health there are innumerable variables or differences in individual body chemistry, absorption rates, reactions, etc., and even these factors change within the same body, so it can be extremely difficult in many cases to find the exact medicine or therapy that works for each individual person.

But it is this fact that each body is so different that makes whole, natural urine so tremendously valuable as a medicine.

Scientists have discovered that urine contains thousands of elements that are specifically related to almost every function of each individual body:

> *"Urine has been referred to as a mirror which reflects the activities within the individual's body ... urine provides information about the functions of the whole body."*

> **— Urinalysis in Clinical and Laboratory Practice**

When you use your own urine medicinally, you get the protein or antibody or hormone, etc., in the correct concentration and structure that your own body has manufactured to regulate itself or to respond to a health threat.

And each of these medically important elements is in a perfect and immensely complex interrelationship with thousands of other important urine components. But this vital relationship of natural components is completely lost when we extract separate urine ingredients for medical use.

Medical researchers want to extract these valuable urine components so that they can convert them into drug products that can be mass-marketed to consumers.

But commercially produced urine extracts are not comparable to your own urine because your urine contains elements that reflect and treat your precise health condition and body functions – and these elements are too complex to be duplicated in an extract or drug.

For instance, as this next newspaper article reveals, researchers have been trying extract an ingredient from urine that has been proven to promote healthy sleep so they can use it in drug form:

FACTOR S:
Help for the Wee, Wee Hours

A MYSTERIOUS biochemical substance that safely and naturally induces deep sleep has been found in human urine.

Dubbed "Factor S" by the scientists at Harvard University and the University of Chicago, the substance has proved to be especially effective as a promoter of healthy sleep...

Extensive trials of the biochemical are continuing but it is expected to take some years before a commercially produced version of Factor S will be available to the public.

Now this article would have us believe that we can't utilize the benefits of Factor S until a commercially produced 'drug version' is made available to the public. But as urine therapy research shows, we can use urine in its natural form and experience its amazing benefits without waiting for a drug version or exposing ourselves to drug side effects.

And there are important reasons why we should use natural urine therapy rather than urine extracts or synthetic drug forms.

For instance, let's suppose that researchers do successfully produce a "Factor S" drug and that you're suffering from sleeplessness. You go to your doctor and are given the drug so you'll sleep better. But what you and the doctor don't know is that your insomnia is caused by an undiagnosed food allergy which isn't cured by taking the sleep drug. You take the drug for a few weeks, but now you're having side effects – headaches, dizziness and drowsiness during the day. So you stop taking the Factor S drug.

But as soon as you stop taking the drug, your sleeping disorder comes back, because the allergy that's causing the insomnia has never been identified or treated.

If you had used natural urine therapy in this scenario, rather than the Factor S drug, you could have been treating and healing your undiagnosed allergy because your urine contained the exact antibody needed to overcome the food allergy, and at the same time, you'd have solved your sleep disorder because the allergy that caused it had been eliminated – all at no cost and without the danger of side effects.

When we use only one component of urine or of any natural medicinal substance, we miss the often extraordinary benefits of all the other ingredients.

Even some medical doctors themselves are now questioning the wisdom of using just one extracted ingredient of a natural substance rather than the natural substance itself in treating disease. Dr. Andrew Weil, M.D., is a noted and certified American physician with a strong background on the use of natural medicinal plants in healing, who now utilizes natural plants in treating his own patients.

Dr. Weil has observed in his own research and practice that it is safer and often more effective to use a natural plant treatment rather than a refined derivative of the plant. He has observed, as have many other doctors, that isolated extracts are generally more toxic than their natural sources and sometimes even fail to give the same medical benefits as the natural sources they're derived from:

> *"In their enthusiasm at isolating the active principles of drug plants, researchers made a serious mistake. They came to believe that all of a plant's desirable properties could be accounted for by a single compound...The erroneous idea that plants and isolated active principles are equivalent has become fixed dogma in pharmacology and medicine...[but] purified drugs are not the same as the plants they come from."*

— The Value of Using Whole Plants Health and Healing

Another good example of why whole urine is a more desirable medicine than urine extracts is shown by research discoveries done on urea, the principal solid ingredient of urine.

Researchers discovered almost one hundred years ago that concentrated urea itself can destroy many different strains of disease bacteria and viruses but seemed less effective on certain other bacterial strains, such as tuberculosis. But even though urea is less effective in killing TB, in the 1950's, research proved that whole urine has been shown to rapidly and in many cases, completely inhibit and destroy the TB bacteria!

One of the unfortunate things about this story is that the researcher who discovered urine's anti-TB properties, rather than announcing that urine could essentially cure TB, instead spent years unsuccessfully trying to identify and isolate the urine component that killed the TB bacteria so that a drug could be formulated from it.

You might think that in this day of modern antibiotics, TB isn't a relevant issue, but it is:

TUBERCULOSIS ON RISE IN U.S.
The Associated Press
Friday, October 8, 1993

WASHINGTON – New cases of tuberculosis are increasing at an alarming rate...congressional analysts reported Thursday.

"This is a chilling report; it is an indictment of our public-health system," said Rep. Ed Towns, D-N.Y., chairman of the House Governmental Operations subcommittee on human resources...

The congressional report said efforts to combat tuberculosis is complicated because of the emergence of strains resistant to anti-TB drugs..."

A recent article in a doctor's publication also revealed that TB has now increased at an alarming rate among children, and is even causing fatalities, because the disease strikes children much harder than adults. And doctors are finding it extremely difficult to deal with this new TB epidemic because it's easily misdiagnosed and is now resistant to anti-TB drugs.

— American Medical News
Feb. 14, 1994

Isolating separate elements from natural substances and refining or chemically copying them as synthetic drug forms isn't the miracle technique that modern medical science would have us believe. Scientists and doctors throughout the twentieth century taught consumers that purified and refined isolated extracts were far more effective and just as safe as the natural substances they were derived from, but time has proven them wrong.

Not only are hundreds of the drugs we routinely use everyday unproven and potentially dangerous, but this continual drug-taking also interferes with our body's ability to develop natural immunity to disease.

As the article on TB and others like it reveal, bacteria are successfully adapting to our drugs, but obviously, our immune systems haven't developed immunity to the bacteria, because we've relentlessly overridden our natural immune responses and functions with chemical drugs. Now the drugs don't work – so where does that leave us? It leaves us, by all accounts, in serious trouble.

A recent report from the Centers For Disease Control (CDC) stated that in U.S. hospitals, a major disease-causing bacterium has now become resistant to antibiotics normally used to treat infected patients:

> *In 1992, CDC reported that more than 2 million patients annually suffer from infections; in 1992, 19,027 people died from infections contracted in the hospital, and another 58,092 died from causes to which such infections had contributed.*

— Associated Press

There is no doubt that drugs and surgery do play a part in medicine, but these therapies have their limitations, even in treating serious infectious diseases. Strong synthetic drugs have no place in the everyday health armamentarium of consumers. The only real reason why we and our doctors now unthinkingly and routinely overuse drugs and surgery is because they are so heavily promoted by the drug industry which makes billions of dollars each year from these methods.

But you don't have to throw away your hard-earned money on unsafe, inappropriate drugs and put your health at risk with chemical drugs or surgery in order to get well.

As many doctors themselves now believe, traditional natural medical methods like urine therapy are completely valid should play a prominent part in our personal health treatments and preventive health care.

Does The Doctor Really Know Best?

If you still feel apprehensive about trying urine therapy because your doctor doesn't recommend it, consider what conventional doctors really do know about real healing – even when they use their own conventional medical techniques.

In his book, What Your Doctor Didn't Learn in Medical School...and what you can do about it!, Dr. Stuart M. Berger, M.D. tells about the fallacies and flaws in our medical school regimens and teaching practices.

Dr. Berger tells about his medical apprenticeship at Tufts Medical School, Harvard School of Public Health and New York's prestigious University Hospital, where he and his classmates had access to the most sophisticated space-age medical technologies available, including masterful surgical techniques that seem to defy death.

> *"We were learning immense amounts"* says Dr. Berger, *"but were we learning what we should? We were becoming doctors, to be sure, but were we becoming better healers?"*

Later in his life, when Dr. Berger's mother was nearly killed by a mistaken cancer diagnosis, he witnessed first-hand the often fatal breakdown of the medical system under which he and all allopathic doctors are trained. As Dr. Berger tells us, his mother's life, but for his intervention, might have been lost because of her doctors' mismanagement:

> *"She had come only days away from being pumped full of the most lethal, debilitating agents – **drugs quite capable of crippling or even killing her, for a cancer she never had...***
>
> *Her life could have been forfeited to delay, mismanagement, [and] the needless toxic interventions of a medical system run amok.*
>
> *I also know that the same is true of every man, woman and child who participates in our medical system – and that means all of us. This sorry state of things is a simple fact of American medicine, one that holds true for you, for your loved ones and for your friends.*

The truth is that we are all at risk simply because of how our medical system functions. Or, to put it another way, because of what our doctors didn't learn in medical school."

Like many other conscientious doctors today, Berger urges everyone to become informed consumers. Just as Berger and thousands of us have experienced – your life may depend on what you, not your doctors, know about medical therapies and your own body.

Another good book on the perils of modern medicine is *Medicine on Trial* by Charles Inlander, Lowell Levin and Ed Weiner. Lowell Levin is a professor at Yale University School of Medicine:

"Twelve of the thirteen chapters in this book are devoted exclusively to evidence of misconduct and mayhem perpetrated on an unsuspecting public [by the medical profession]. 'Serious' is too tame a word...One has to wonder why the facts presented in this book have not heretofore been put on public view forcefully.

Why has the honorable profession of medicine kept the facts of its mistakes to itself? Is the profession of medicine so venal that it is willing to risk the lives of people whose trust it enjoys? Can the [medical] profession and its institutions be so cynical as to treat patients and the public at large as incapable of understanding what is going on?

People sense that physicians may not be the omniscient and totally dedicated care givers that organized medicine's image makers have been advertising. Personal experiences of family and friends drive home the reality of medicine's clay feet.

There are growing signs that the public has had enough cover-up and outright deceit. People are not fools, even though they may have been fooled, or more likely, lulled, into believing that medical care has been on a steady course of progress, from one medical miracle to another. The overselling and hype about winning the war on cancer is an example...We have been fed a considerable number of public relations releases about medicine's successes, with little or no effort to portray its downside.

Government studies now raise questions about the qualifications (or lack thereof) of physicians...their misdiagnoses, unnecessary or incompetent surgery, errors in medication, neglect and high hospital infection rates... Money, power, prestige and egos conspire to hold reformists [inside the medical system] to marginal, largely cosmetic changes."

Anyone who is currently taking any doctor-recommended and supposedly therapeutic drug of any type also needs to read the book, *The Informed Consumer's Pharmacy, The Essential Guide to Prescription and Over-the-Counter Drugs* by Ellen Hodgson Brown and Lynne Paige Walker. This book is one of the clearest, most comprehensive guides to therapeutic drugs available, and if you value your good health, you'll definitely want to read it.

As the authors of *The Informed Consumer's Pharmacy* comment:

> *"Overdosing on drugs is the most popular form of suicide, but drugs in lesser amounts can kill as surely. Like time bombs, they just act more slowly. **More Americans are killed each year by drugs than by auto accidents.** The American Medical Association estimates as much as one-third of all illness may be 'iatrogenic' — caused by drugs and other medical therapies aimed at a cure.*
>
> *It has also been estimated that 70-80 percent of the people who visit doctors have nothing wrong with them that wouldn't be cleared up by a vacation, a raise, or relief from the stresses of their lives. Another 10 percent have diseases for which there is no cure. Only 10 percent would benefit from drugs or surgery. Yet 57 percent or more come away with prescriptions."*

The New York Times Medical Science section on August 17, 1993, reported that new research findings show that as many as two-thirds of patients who are treated with placebos for health complaints improve after taking the placebo — that's twice as many patients as originally calculated by researchers testing new drugs.

A placebo is a sugar-pill or a drug that has no objective effect on the symptoms being treated. One doctor quoted in the article suggests that all doctors should start using the placebo effect to their advantage by giving patients drugs even though the doctor does not know what the patient's illness is, or if the patient is actually sick at all: "If a doctor believes in what he's doing and lets the patient know that, that's good medicine."

Studies show that the majority of Americans today are so convinced that their "doctors know better" that they get better even when the drug substance they're given has nothing to do with treating the disorder they're suffering from.

So, in essence, your doctor may have selected an unnecessary or incorrect drug for you to take, but you get better because psychologically you feel you should.

Unfortunately, the health improvement may be imaginary, but the side effects of the drug that show up later won't be:

> *"...However drugs are produced and distributed, a separate and equally important issue is how doctors prescribe them. As noted, physicians prescribe largely on the basis of information from drug houses. If the packaging and copy are effective and persistent enough, the physician will probably prescribe the product...*
>
> *[But] the disregard of contraindications for the use of drugs causes thousands of unnecessary illnesses every year."*

— Betrayal of Health

Every medicine we use does not have to be synthesized and commercially produced in order to be effective and safe. And, as we've seen, drugs and surgery are the last forms of medicine that we should resort to, and not the first choice, as they are for the majority of us today.

As Hippocrates taught, *nature first* is the best health regimen. We all need to give common sense health care and non-invasive medicines an informed chance before we rush into dangerous chemical or surgical therapies that can create more symptoms and problems than they relieve.

And many people are learning to think for themselves and not to take their doctors bad advice lying down, as a recent article in *The Wall Street Journal*, June 16, 1993, demonstrates:

> *"Al Iglehart figures his doctors pegged him for a fool.*
>
> *They knew his heart disease was congenital, without mysterious complications. Still, they suggested he undergo more tests, even repeat a $1200 one he had already passed. Thank you for the advice, Mr. Iglehart said. But absolutely not.*
>
> *'The doctor just isn't God, and sometimes they're on autopilot,' says Mr Iglehart, who is 44 years old and live on Long Island, N.Y. 'There was no reason for any more tests. The biggest thing you can do [about medical treatments] is to be informed as a consumer and ask questions.'*
>
> *Mr. Iglehart is among a growing group of defiant health-care patients who are questioning the costs [and effectiveness] of medical procedures..."*

It isn't my intention to go into a lot of 'doctor-bashing' here, because doctors, of course, play a crucial role in medicine, but they have assumed, and we have given them an impossible role and responsibility in medicine today. We expect our doctors to behave like mechanics, to diagnose and to fix every possible thing that goes wrong with us, as if our bodies were cars or machines that could be repaired simply by pouring in some synthetic substance or replacing a part.

But our bodies aren't machines, and our doctors should be relieved of their role as mechanics that we run to every time we feel sick. Our bodies are immensely intricate, sensitive, individually unique, living organisms that need gentle respect and care, not the incessant and routine overkill of concentrated drugs and invasive surgery.

Doctors can certainly play an important role in urine therapy, especially in acute illnesses where injections of urea or urine could be life saving, as is clearly seen in one of the research studies in which intravenous urea saved the life of a patient with severe cerebral edema caused by a brain tumor (see next chapter). Also, natural urine therapy could most definitely be enhanced and augmented by doctors' administrations of natural urine extracts or urea for serious illnesses.

However, for most illnesses, we can treat ourselves with natural urine therapy and save our valuable doctors precious time and effort.

Learning to Care for Our Own Health

Unfortunately, today's consumers have been exposed to the most intensive media advertising barrage in the history of medicine, and are now conditioned to expect medicines and health therapies to deliver an instantaneous "punch" – irregardless of the cost, side effects or ultimate consequences of such methods.

If we get headaches, rather than getting more rest or eliminating the three chocolate bars and Coke we had for lunch, we 'whomp' our bodies with the strongest headache medicine we can buy – never mind that the infinitesimally small type on the label lists twenty different serious side effects of the drug.

Many people have complained to me over the years that they've tried homeopathy or herbs or other types of natural healing instead of drugs with no success. But when we examine their situation in depth, I invariably find that they were trying to use natural therapies in the same way that they use drugs – popping a pill from a bottle they picked up on a health food store shelf and waiting for a quick fix, or drinking a cup or two of herbal tea and then deciding, "Nope, don't feel better – didn't work for me."

But the problem is not the natural medicines, the problem is the approach.

The simple fact is that no matter what medicines we take or health therapies we try, natural or synthetic, if we don't change our overall bad health habits and lifestyles we aren't going to be healthy and we aren't going to feel good.

In order for natural therapies to work, you really have to begin to get in touch with what the requirements of good health really are. Real and lasting physical health is based on much more than continually knocking out unpleasant symptoms with medicines or surgery.

A nutritious diet, rest, relaxation, exercise, a healthy living environment and a balanced, positive, peaceful and happy frame of mind are the indispensable foundations of good and lasting health. When you improve your basic health habits by incorporating these elements into your daily lifestyle, you enhance your natural immune defenses and improve your health and ability to fight disease.

Natural medicines can be used, when necessary, in order to augment your healing if and when you do happen to get sick; this combination of a strong natural immunity and gentle, immune-strengthening natural medicinals is the best possible solution to our health problems.

Trying to achieve good health by routinely using drugs and surgery to suppress disease symptoms produced by unhealthy lifestyles is a dead end – literally.

Just because the generally accepted modern lifestyle has conditioned us to believe and accept that McDonald's is really a place to eat and that white sugar is a nutritive food, isn't going to change the fact that neither of those things is true. As doctors tell us:

> *"Today's chronic diseases – both social and medical – are really symptoms of a much more vast underlying problem. They are the culmination of years of inadequate nutrition, a toxic environment, sedentary lifestyles, familial and social disruptions, and dependence on artificial agents (from cigarettes to cocaine) for happiness. Every cell in our bodies – from the brain to the immune system – is affected by these abuses."*
> **— Betrayal of Health**

You can't halfheartedly lay a veneer of natural medicines over your inherently unhealthy and destructive lifestyle and then announce to yourself and the world that you tried natural medicine and "it didn't work."

Everyday as a nation we consumers drink millions of gallons of those toxic brews called Pepsi and Coke; we ingest millions of dollars worth of junk food, food additives and sugar, stuffing it all down at warp speed as we madly propel ourselves through overcrowded streets in cars belching carbon monoxide fumes, all the while breathing in the toxic aroma of the grossly polluted air.

Arriving at our synthetically constructed domiciles, we subject our bodies and minds to relentless TV radiation and the dismal harangue of the nightly news, all the while "banging" our stress and sugar induced headaches, aches and pains with Bayer, or Excedrin, Anacin or Dristan, or whatever other 'wonder drug' flashes seductively across the screen.

And then we ask ourselves "Why don't I feel good – why can't my doctor fix me once and for all?

Because of our modern lifestyle, too few of us pause to rest and treat our bodies with love, caring or respect. When we go to the drugstore, our only thought is to find the fastest-acting, strongest drug available to relieve our discomfort and in essence, to 'shut the body up'. And drug companies and doctors know this – so they give us what we think we want, and what we erroneously assume is safe.

So how do we start looking out for our own health concerns? We can start by not rushing to the drugstore or doctor for a quick-fix every time we don't feel well. We can change our lifestyles and we can learn how to gently stimulate our immune defenses, treat illness and relieve pain with simple natural medicines like urine therapy.

And we can change our diets. It's not that hard to get back to simple basics – get rid of the frozen and boxed dinners, the instant breakfast shakes, the sodas, the sugary, preservative, chemical-filled desserts and start eating real foods like whole grains and fresh green vegetables and salads and fruit. Our environment is so filled with chemical pollutants today that deliberately ingesting them in our food is an unwise practice and an added burden on our already overburdened immune systems.

The use of basic natural foods and natural medicines, unlike synthetic drugs or surgery, requires a degree of self-love, self-discipline, and patience – listening to the body, observing the causes behind the symptoms of our illnesses, and changing unhealthy habits and attitudes, rather than relying on strong medical interventions to mask underlying disease factors by relieving symptoms.

No matter how inconvenient these changes might seem now, just wait until you see how inconvenient cancer, heart disease and serious chronic illness can be if you don't make these changes.

So as you can see, there is a chain of command within our present medical system that has made it difficult, or nearly impossible for the research information and findings on simple, inexpensive urine therapy to receive recognition:

1) Getting FDA approval for medical therapies is astronomically expensive;

2) Drug companies want high-profit, patentable therapies to pay for research and to boost company profits;

3) Hospitals and doctors are indoctrinated and influenced by heavy promotion and pressure from the pharmaceutical industry, and so prescribe and use only drug company endorsed medical therapies.

A New Era in Medicine

Fortunately, attitudes in medicine are changing in response to the many problems that have surfaced with drug and surgical therapies. Recent articles show the general trend by both consumers and the medical community towards traditional, more natural health approaches. A study cited recently in the *New England Journal of Medicine* stated that:

> *In 1990, Americans made 425 million visits to alternative health care practitioners, while 388 million visits were made to conventional health care providers.*

> **— Focus on Behavioral Health Magazine**
> **July 9, 1993**

Another article in *Forbes Magazine*, reports on the new trend in medicine back to traditional, natural forms of healing:

"New Support for Old Therapies"

"Does the doctor really know best? Not always, it would seem, if you take into account the increasing respectability being won by such non-

conventional therapies as acupuncture, biofeedback, chiropractic and herbal medicine.

In other cultures these therapies have been standard practice for ages, but most physicians educated in schools approved by the American Medical Association and affiliated with AMA hospitals have long dismissed these techniques as quackery.

Today, however, signs of a new approbation for alternative medicine are everywhere. Even The National Institutes of Health now has an Office of Alternative Medicine."

— Forbes, Dec. 20, 1993

It's interesting to realize how much power we consumers have over our own lives. As this article demonstrates, individual consumers are the ones who can ultimately determine the course of medicine over the next century by the choices they make for medical treatments. And the medical establishment knows this, as another recent article reveals:

The National Institutes of Health Begins a New Era...

For the first time, it will systematically explore unconventional medical practices, decide which are effective and begin putting some of them into mainstream medicine.

Stephen Groft, who heads the new effort, said a panel of experts will study many methods long scoffed at by traditional doctors, including acupuncture, naturopathy, homeopathy, Ayurvedic medicine, reflexology, massage therapy and Chinese herbal remedies."

Sounds like good news, doesn't it? Unfortunately, though, these time-honored proven natural methods are going to have to somehow be made to fit the modern scientific medical model – one which has already been shown to have largely failed:

"Many scientists are actually excited to see that alternative methods are being scientifically evaluated,' Groft said. 'It is important to separate those that are working from those that aren't working – for both patients and physicians...

The task is to assess the scientific evidence already available, determine whether more research is worthwhile and give priority to funding."

— Gannett News Service
August, 1993

Sound familiar? It's the same old strains of the same old song – we, the scientific "experts" will tell you what works for you. But we've already examined where their 'proof' comes from and just how unreliable it is. Ironically, the agency that is calling for scientific evaluation of these natural health treatments is The National Institutes of Health that was itself responsible for the recent tests on the hepatitis drug that killed nearly all of the research participants. So just how valuable are the medical community's 'scientific' assessments?

At this point in time, we need to stop examining and picking apart therapies that have hundreds, and in some cases, thousands of years of practical experience behind them. Rather than wasting their time and our money on the unnecessary contortions of trying to "scientifically" prove what hundreds of thousands of patients have already experienced over many centuries with these simple and safe natural techniques, the National Institutes of Health and their panel of experts' efforts would be infinitely better spent on deciding how to formulate new and inexpensive FDA guidelines for approving traditional medical therapies and in qualifying responsible health care practitioners for both conventional and natural medicine.

This simple adjustment alone could tremendously reduce health care costs and dramatically upgrade health care quality by providing and teaching effective, simple, inexpensive natural medical self-help approaches like urine therapy that can take the place of expensive and dangerous drugs and surgical therapies that should be rightly reserved for crisis and emergency care, and free up doctors' and specialists' precious time.

We already know that traditional natural therapies like herbal medicines, urine therapy and homeopathy work, and many are still widely used in other civilized countries. Chinese hospitals and doctors even today largely depend on their traditional natural herbal medicine and acupuncture; England has homeopathic hospitals; Germans rely heavily on their herbal medicines which are even available in their drugstores. In France, too, pharmacies carry and doctors prescribe natural homeopathic and herbal medicines in addition to synthetic drugs.

There are a wonderful variety of alternatives to invasive and synthetic medicine that have been proven to be safe and effective over centuries of use and observations, we just have to relearn the art of using them and cure ourselves of our dependency on drugs and surgery. Also, there are many more books *(see Appendix)* besides the ones I've already mentioned in this chapter which will help you to learn more about how to care for your health safely and effectively.

The challenge of achieving and maintaining good health is in creating a balanced lifestyle and in finding the combination of natural treatments and remedies that are right for you individually.

And as you'll discover in this book, urine therapy is the most powerful, most individualized natural medicine we could ever hope for. After reading all that urine therapy has to offer, I know you'll agree that even though man has failed to find the synthetic "magic bullet" medicine to cure every illness, Nature had already created it for us and given us an incredible, safe, cost-free and simple, natural tool to heal ourselves – our body's own amazing, natural medicine.

CHAPTER 4

THE RESEARCH EVIDENCE AND CASE STUDIES

The medical applications of urine and its constituents have been tested, discussed, researched and utilized to such an extent throughout the twentieth century that it seems incredible that almost none of us, including the majority of our doctors and medical administrators have ever heard anything about it.

But again, the reason for this is not entirely a mystery. As we discussed in the last chapter, even though the success of urine therapy was reported long before the 1900's, twentieth century medical researchers, doctors and the public were no longer interested in traditional natural medicines.

So urine therapy was moved out of the home and doctor's offices and into the oblivion of research laboratories, where, unfortunately, it still largely remains today.

As we've discussed, urine therapy largely disappeared from public use at the turn of the century and the knowledge of the therapy is now hidden in medical journals and research reports that people and doctors in general never see; also, urine ingredients are simply isolated and converted into unrecognizable drug forms.

Even though there have been amazing scientific discoveries about the medical use of urine, medical researchers, for the most part, do not tell the public about their discoveries. Again, this situation is most likely the result of two factors. One, modern medical researchers are primarily oriented towards finding strong, monetarily profitable chemical "bullets" to knock out specific diseases – and not towards discovering natural medicines which augment the body's natural capacity to heal.

Secondly, most medical researchers work for pharmaceutical companies and many are contractually bound not to reveal the results of their research until the research can be applied as a profit-making medical therapy that can be patented by the company who funded the research.

Also, medical researchers tend to devote their research to extremely specialized branches of medicine, and these separate departments of medicine don't generally communicate their findings to departments outside of their own research fields. So the urologists, for instance, who discovered that urine can prevent and heal urinary tract infections might publish their findings for other urologists, but a doctor in general practice would probably not come in contact with these studies on the importance of urine in bladder or kidney infections.

The public and most practicing doctors today consider urine to be nothing more than a body waste. But many medical researchers know that in reality, urine is an enormously comprehensive and powerful medical substance. Now you get to read what many scientists and doctors know, but haven't told us about the amazing curative effects of urine therapy.

The research studies and articles selected for this chapter are each numbered and presented in chronological order to present a broad overview of how consistently and intensively urine has been researched during the twentieth century.

You'll be amazed and astounded by these studies on the medical use of urine. As I was reading over these reports, and looking at all of the other many studies on urine therapy, I couldn't help exclaiming "Why didn't anyone ever tell us?".

More About Urea

As an added note, many of these research studies were done using the urine extract, urea, which is the primary organic solid of urine. Urea, an organic salt formed in the liver, is the result of the body's use, or synthesis, of protein. The body eliminates excess nitrogen which is produced during protein metabolism in the form of urea. Urea is also used by the body to help in the mechanism which determines how concentrated the urine is, or in other words, how much water is excreted from the blood. Urea was discovered centuries ago, in 1773, when it was first separated from urine; later, in 1828, natural urea was synthesized or chemically "copied" in the laboratory.

The discovery of urea was one of the most important events of modern chemistry and biochemistry because it was the first organic compound to be separated in a relatively pure state. Urea, which is critical to our body's use of protein, also provides innumerable profound keys as to how our bodies work and function.

For this reason, chemists have been fascinated for years by urea and its amazing and diverse applications in the fields of science and medicine:

> *"More scientific papers have probably been published on urea than on any other organic compound..."*
> — **Journal of the American Medical Association**
>   **July 1954, "De Urina"**

Urea has so many beneficial properties that it was used historically, and is still used today, in a wide variety of medical applications – for reducing excess fluid pressure on the brain, as a remarkable skin treatment for eczema, dry skin disorders, and fungal infections; as a moisturizer in cosmetic creams, as a safe and effective diuretic, and as an anti-bacterial, antiseptic treatment for healing serious wounds.

People who have heard of the term "uremia", or uremic poisoning, often assume that urea itself is toxic and is therefore excreted in the urine. But this is not the case. Excess urea becomes toxic to the body only when the filtering mechanisms of the kidneys are damaged or impaired, and the urea level of the blood is not properly regulated But in this case, excessive amounts of other benign substances like water and sodium become toxic also if the kidney is unable to regulate them in the blood. As you'll discover in the research studies in this chapter, urea is not only not toxic, but in reality has tremendous medical and physiological value, and can be safely used even in large quantities.

Urea is on the FDA list of approved drugs for medical use and many products made from urea are listed in the Physician's Desk Reference, (which is the book that doctors refer to in deciding what drug to prescribe), and in the *U.S. Pharmacological Index.*

However, as wonderful as urea has proven to be in medicine, I want to stress that it cannot and should not be used to replace or supersede natural urine as a healing agent. As the research in this chapter proves, whole urine contains hundreds of known and unknown medically important elements that clearly and definitively are not found in urea alone.

Also, as medical studies have unequivocally shown, each person's urine contains antibodies, natural 'vaccines' and many other critical physiological elements that are carried in the blood that are specific to each individual's health condition. These elements in whole urine are not found in either natural or synthetic urea alone.

For instance, if you have an allergic reaction to wheat, your body produces a complex of antibodies to deal with the allergy and those antibodies are found in your urine. Medical studies have demonstrated that when you reintroduce these urine antibodies into your system by ingesting or injecting your own urine, that the allergy can be corrected. But urea alone would not contain these allergy-fighting antibodies.

In using your own urine to heal yourself, you're getting medicinal elements that your particular body has produced in order to deal with your specific, intricate and often undetectable disturbances in your body's functioning.

You could be exposed to polio, for example or tuberculosis and not even realize it until acute symptoms appear – but, as medical research has proven, your urine can contain antibodies to those diseases even if acute symptoms are not appearing. So regular use of urine therapy can most definitely provide extremely comprehensive therapeutic treatment that goes far beyond urea or other medicines.

This is not to say that other therapies are not useful and effective, they are, of course, but urine therapy, correctly applied, should be the foundation for our health regimens and medical treatments and should definitely be used routinely in illness and preventive health care.

I recently read a magazine article about a 12 year-old girl in the Midwest who was admitted to the hospital with a high fever, lassitude, and drooling heavily from the mouth. Doctors tried frantically but unsuccessfully to diagnose her condition but she deteriorated and died several days later. Only after her death was it discovered that she'd died of an undiagnosed and therefore untreated case of rabies.

This is a good example of why urine and urea therapy should be incorporated into all types of medicine. In this girl's case, urine therapy could have been invaluable. In the first place, urea itself has been scientifically proven to dissolve or destroy the rabies virus, so it could most definitely have aided this little girl.

Additionally, the rabies antibody would have been present in the girl's urine, so she would have gotten the benefit of both the urea and the rabies antibody after ingesting her urine. Her doctors couldn't diagnose her illness – but her body already had, and if she'd been given her urine orally, or by injection with perhaps, added urea, it might well have saved her life.

And the real tragedy is that there is absolutely no downside risk here – absolutely none!. Urine is free, it's backed by almost 100 years of medical testing, and in every single study ever done on urine and urea's medicinal use in humans, no toxicity has ever been reported. So what did this young girl have to lose by being treated with them?

As hundreds of people have experienced, and as research has shown, urine is undoubtedly an amazing natural medicine that can give you health benefits beyond any other natural or chemical substance in existence.

The information on the medical uses of urine most definitely deserves public recognition and frankly, if we don't routinely take advantage of this incredible natural remedy, we can't honestly say that we're doing all that we can to preserve and regain our good health.

Sometimes it's hard to believe that even with all our medical knowledge and technological genius, we still don't have strong, healthy, disease-resistant bodies – but the fact that widespread, crippling health disorders still abound should tell us that we're doing something wrong and overlooking something important.

Let's not overlook this simplest and yet most useful of natural medicines.

RESEARCH AND CLINICAL STUDIES

Report #1

TITLE: *PLEOMORPHISM, AS EXHIBITED BY BACTERIA GROWN ON A MEDIA CONTAINING UREA,* 1906, by W. James Wilson, B.A., M.B, from the Pathological Laboratory of Queen's College Belfast, published in the Journal of Pathological Bacteria, London.

SUBJECT: *THE ANTI-BACTERIAL EFFECT OF UREA*

This laboratory study is presented first because it's one of the more thorough and earliest twentieth century laboratory research studies on the medical applications of urea.

Don't be intimidated by the word 'pleomorphism'. In this context it just basically means that urea changed the shape, or stopped the normal growth of disease bacteria.

After medical researchers discovered that certain types of living microorganisms, such as bacteria, could cause disease, it became almost their sole aim to discover ways of killing or stopping the growth of these microorganisms, or germs.

In this particular study, the researcher, James Wilson, placed different disease-causing bacteria, such as Bacillus typhosus (typhoid) into petri dishes containing urea solutions and found, as had other researchers, that the urea stopped the normal growth of the bacteria:

into what?

> *"In October 1905, at the suggestion of Professor Symmers, I was investigating the action of the Bacillus typhosus and the B.Coli on urea. I...found that as the percentage of urea in the medium varied, so did the amount of growth of the bacillus...*
>
> *...with greater percentages of urea, the growth of the organism was inhibited; with 7 per cent (urea), very little growth occurred; with 8 per cent practically none...*
>
> *Urea has an antiseptic or inhibitory effect on the growth of microorganisms."*

This anti-bacterial effect of urea was also proven by several other researchers very early in the twentieth century. But rather than present each of these studies on urea separately, the most notable of these research findings are listed below in order to give a coherent overview on the important studies on urea that were conducted and published during the first decades of the new era of modern medicine:

1900

A German researcher by the name of Spiro reported his discovery that urea solutions have a remarkable ability to "dissolve" foreign proteins. This is medically important because viruses, for example, are molecular proteins as are allergens. Later research confirmed that urea has an amazing ability to rapidly and easily destroy viruses such as polio and rabies viruses, and during the 1980's, urine was defined as an extremely effective treatment for a wide variety of allergies.

1902

W. Ramsden, another researcher, published a report in the American Journal of Physiology further detailing the protein dissolving properties of urea. Ramsden also discovered that urea prevented putrefaction in wounds. His work is often referred to by later researchers looking into the anti-bacterial applications of urea.

1906

Two French researchers, G. Peju and H. Rajat published a report on their detailed study of the effect of urea on various disease-causing bacteria. Their research demonstrated that the more concentrated the urea, the more it inhibited bacterial growth. In concentrated solutions of urea, no bacterial growth occurred. The research done by Peju and Rajat has been referred to many times over the years by other researchers who studied and clinically applied the anti-bacterial properties of urea. This research also supported the later use of urea as an antiseptic in the treatment of wounds and infections during the 1930's and 40's.

1915

In England, two other researchers, W. Symmers and T.S Kirk, published their report entitled "Urea as a Bactericide and Its Application in the Treatment of Wounds". Symmers and Kirk were actually military doctors, so of course their work with urea centered around its use as an antiseptic for wounds.

In their report, they comment that: "all the wounded soldiers under our care in the Ulster Volunteer Force Hospital have been treated with urea, and it has been found that...infected wounds dressed with urea once in 24 hours give better results than similar cases treated in any other way." Later 20th century researchers firmly established and proved that urea, both topically, and internally, provides a wide variety of excellent benefits and produces no adverse side effects.

As you read more about the remarkable clinical data on the benefits of urea further on, you'll be extremely surprised that our medical community today has failed to emphasize the use of this incredibly inexpensive, effective and safe anti-bacterial medicine.

Report #2

TITLE: *AUTOTHERAPY,* (book), 1918, by Dr. Charles H. Duncan. The following report is taken from a chapter from Dr. Duncan's book entitled *"Urine as An Autotherapeutic Remedy"*. Dr. Duncan was the Attending Surgeon, Genito-Urinary Specialist and co-founder of the Volunteer Hospital, New York City.

Dr. Duncan used the word Autotherapy, as have other doctors, to refer to the utilization of natural substances of the body to create a healing response. In his chapter on "Urine as An Autotherapeutic Remedy," Dr. Duncan describes his clinical observations on the use of urine therapy in his medical practice, and discusses reports from other doctors who were using urine therapy at the time.

From an historical point of view, it's interesting to note the seriousness with which urine therapy was treated by even mainstream twentieth century doctors. Dr. Duncan was a practicing surgeon, founder of the Volunteer Hospital in New York City, a Genito-Urinary Specialist –and a supporter of natural urine therapy.

Our medical community today in general would have us believe that urine therapists are traveling road-show quacks giving out ludicrous and unsubstantiated medical claims, but that's a gross misrepresentation of the truth.

As Dr. Duncan observed:

"There is scarcely a pathogenic (disease) condition which does not affect the urine contents...It may be said that urine is like a weather vane, sensitively registering any change in the patient's condition, be it great or small.

Many pathogenic conditions...are quickly cured by the therapeutic employment of urine alone...it is significant, indeed, when Clark's Materia Medica gives many conditions in which uric acid and urea have been proved to be therapeutically effective.

In the New York Medical Journal of December 14 and 21, 1912 and in the Therapeutic Record of January 1914, I reported that I was employing urine successfully in the treatment of many conditions...since then it has been employed successfully both by myself and many other physicians in treating patients suffering with a great variety of pathogenic conditions."

Duncan goes on to cite several case studies in which he successfully used urine therapy. For instance:

CASE 190.   *"Patient, male, 30 years, applied for treatment for cystitis that developed after a long drive in the rain. At night he had to void every hour or two...A teaspoonful of morning urine one-half hour before* meals completely cleared up the case within two days."

CASE 198.   *"Patient, male, age 50 years, applied for treatment suffering with inflammation of the bladder and prostate...Upon rising from a sitting posture it was necessary to void urine within a minute. He had to get up at night five and six times. The usual remedies for such conditions gave little or no relief. It was then decided to treat him autotherapeutically. He was instructed to take a drachm of early morning urine a half hour before each meal.*

Within twenty-four hours his improved condition was so marked that be became alarmed thinking his recovery was too quick. [He stopped the therapy] and the pain and tenesmus (spasms) returned; he continued the treatment and improved greatly. He gradually improved and he is [now] apparently in good health."

CASE 203.   The following article by Dr. C.G. Moore was republished in the New Albany Medical Herald, February, 1915, from the Archives of Pediatrics:

"I find diabetes mellitus an uncommonly difficult disease for the general practitioner to treat. April 14, 1912, I was called to see a little seven-year-old girl. They gave me a history of her having felt badly for a few days and of having had some fever. On

examining the child I found her to have a temperature of 102 degrees F., but all other findings were negative. In a couple of days they informed me her temperature was normal and she was feeling all right, but she was passing a large (sticky) amount of urine frequently.

Having tried all methods of treatment on several other patients whom I have had within the past few months suffering with glycosuria (sugar in the urine), I decided to try Autotherapy, for I had known cases of icterus (jaundice) which had failed to respond to any medical treatment, but cleared up in a very short time when they were given their own urine to drink.

I gave this little girl three ounces of her own urine three times daily and then examined for the sugar percentage and found that when she was taking the urine, the percentage of sugar dropped, and that when it was withdrawn, the percentage increased. I could also see some improvement in her general condition. She did not urinate so often or so much; did not drink so much water; her skin was more moist, she was not so nervous..."

CASE 202.   From the report of Dr. Deachman of N.Y.: *"Patient, male, 49, was extremely nervous and irritable; he had wandering pains all over his body, headache and general lassitude. He complained a great deal of pain in the lumbar region and in the abdomen.*

He improved on nothing I gave him...microscopic urine examination showed red blood cells, pus cells, renal cells and abundance of calcium oxalate crystals.

The treatment consisted of a twenty minim injection of urine diluted 1 to 100 with distilled water. He improved with this to a certain point but did not entirely recover until I used a less diluted urine, after which he made a prompt recovery. Two months after he recovered a urinalysis showed absence of pus and renal cells and a normal volume of urine.

Dr. Deachman comments:

"These are but a few of the many cases I have successfully treated by this method, the value of which I consider inestimable.

I make this statement after a wide experience in [using urine] in treating many patients suffering with chronic diseases and particularly in the use of urine as an autotherapeutic agent. I am free to say that the results obtained with urine therapy are [far better] than the usual recognized methods."

Dr. Duncan's reports on the use of urine therapy are quite detailed and include many other extensive observations on his and other doctors' clinical treatments and case studies on the effects of both orally and hypodermically administered urine therapy.

TITLE: *THE ANTISEPTIC AND BACTERICIDAL ACTION OF UREA,* 1935, by John H. Foulger, M.D., and Lee Foshay, M.D., *Journal of Laboratory and Clinical Medicine.* From the Departments of Pharmacology and Experimental Bacteriology, University of Cincinnati.

Report #3

The researchers in this study, Foulger and Foshay, found that urea was extremely effective in curing or preventing a wide variety of bacterial infections and, unlike sulfa drugs, which were widely used at the time, had no deleterious side effects:

"...In an account of the action of urea...Ramsden (1902) made the very interesting observation that urea prevents putrefaction...the first detailed study of urea as a bactericide, (destroys bacteria), is that of Peju and Rajat...no great attention was paid to the bactericidal action of urea until Symmers and Kirk (1915), (who) found urea of undoubted value as a wash in the treatment of diphtheria carriers (and) the treatment of wounds. **That urea is innocuous to human tissues was adequately proved.**

...In one case with a chronic staphylococcus blood infection, urea (powder) was sprinkled between the layers of tissue and the wound then closed with sutures. Healing followed with no sign of infection. ... Infected wounds dressed with urea powder gave better results than similar wounds treated by other methods...

Unaware of the work of Symmers and Kirk, one of us (J.F,) selected as material for a clinical study of urea a few cases of **purulent otitis media (middle ear infection)...all of the cases which had failed to respond to other local medicaments responded to urea...**

...A boy of ten developed otitis media and **hemorrhagic nephritis (kidney inflammation)** *about the third week of hospitalization for*

scarlet fever...urea treatments were started. The ear discharges at once became less foul...At the same time the blood gradually disappeared from the urine...

The results so far obtained suggest that urea may be of considerable value in the treatment of purulent discharges of many types and in the treatment, also of suppurating wounds producing foul odors. This latter use of urea has been reported recently by Millar (see next report)...

The cheapness and harmlessness of urea should encourage other investigations of its clinical use.

As an added note, Foulger and Foshay also discovered, as did other urea researchers later, that destroying strong bacterial strains such as those which cause staph and strep infections required longer exposure to urea than some other types of bacteria, which is something to keep in mind when using urine therapy to combat staph and strep infections.

Report #4

TITLE: *UREA CRYSTALS IN CANCER,* 1933, by Dr. William M. Millar, From the Department of Surgery, College of Medicine of the University of Cincinnati.

SUBJECT: *USE OF UREA CRYSTALS IN TREATING CANCEROUS LESIONS*

Following Foulger's and Foshay's work on the antibacterial action of urea, Dr. Millar began using urea crystals to heal external cancerous ulcerations:

"The peculiarly penetrating odor of a sloughing cancer is one of the horrible aspects of this disease. For the past year at the Tumor Clinic of the Cincinnati General Hospital, urea crystals have been advocated and prescribed in such cases. If they are packed into the wound, the odor will be stopped to a great extent.

Although they dissolve in a few minutes, the offensive character of the ulcer becomes less with each application.

The crystals are cheap, they possess a considerable antiseptic value, and there is no fear of a systemic reaction..."

As research progressed through the twentieth century, the antibacterial properties of urea became increasingly well-known and it was used in the treatment of wounds and infections in Europe and the U.S. until the development of antibiotic creams in the latter half of the century, when it appears that its antiseptic use was discontinued in favor of the newer and supposedly more effective drugs.

Urea, or urine, is cheap, effective and, as a natural substance, causes no adverse reactions in the body. It's proven antibacterial properties make it an excellent treatment for wounds and burns of all kinds.

TITLE: *AUTO-URINE THERAPY,* 1934, by Dr. Martin Krebs, (pediatrician), from a lecture delivered at the Society of Pediatricians, Leipzig.   *Report #5*

Dr. Krebs, a practicing pediatrician in Dresden, like other many other physicians, was intrigued by reports of the medical uses of patients' own urine to treat and cure a wide variety of disorders. Like Dr. Duncan and other practitioners, he referred to this practice as auto-urine therapy.

Dr. Krebs began injecting urine in the course of his own medical practice and was surprised at the rapid and often extraordinary response:

> *"Through intramuscular injections of the patient's own urine, allergies and certain spastic conditions in children are remarkably improved. Extraordinary improvement can be seen with asthma and hayfever. The use of auto-urine therapy is also indicated in the treatment of muscular spasms caused by birth traumas to the brain.*
>
> *I treated an eight-year old boy with hay-fever by injecting 5 cc. of his own urine, and was surprised at the result. The boy immediately began breathing better, and in a few minutes the extreme redness of the eyes disappeared. Another child who had spent 3 1/2 months in a sanatorium for treatment of his asthma, received an injection of 4 cc. of urine. After only 6 minutes, he was able to breathe deeply and then slept well.*
>
> *After my first experiences with the therapy, I was encouraged to try it on other types of cases, and subsequently treated a 10 month old child who had exhibited partial paralysis and muscle spasms apparently caused by birth trauma. After the first injection of urine, he began to loosen and open his fists, his general movements were freer and he laughed, something which his parents had never seen him do. Also, the attacks of angina which he had experienced, stopped after the injection.*

Urine therapy has been indicated as a treatment for:

1) *toxemia in pregnancy,*
2) *allergic conditions,*
3) *pertussis,*
4) *spasms*
5) *increasing breast milk*
6) *hayfever*
7) *asthma*
8) *migraine-like conditions*
9) *eczema*

I believe that Auto-Urine Therapy is worthy of being applied in the area of pediatric medicine. I highly recommend the therapy in the treatment of hayfever and asthma, and I would like to see further follow-up clinical studies done on its application to the other conditions that were mentioned."

Dr. Krebs undertook further clinical research studies in 1940 using natural urine in treating children. His study, entitled The Use of Convalescent Urine in the Mitigation of Acute Infections, demonstrated that urine therapy (administered by means of enemas) was safe and effective for treating childhood infections such as whooping cough, measles and chicken pox.

Dr. Krebs was impressed by the results of his treatments on 58 infected children, and recommended urine therapy to other physicians as a treatment for infections in children.

Krebs, like many other doctors and researchers, discovered excellent uses for urine therapy and he instructed some of the parents of his young patients how to use it at home for treating their children.

TITLE: *AUTO-URINE VACCINE THERAPY FOR ACUTE HEMOR-RHAGIC NEPHRITIS,* 1934, by Dr. R. Tiberi, Institute of Clinical Medicine, University of Perugia, Italy.

Nephritis is an acute or chronic inflammation of the kidney or in other words, a kidney infection, which can be a serious health threat and is difficult to cure. The kidneys are essential for maintaining proper nutrient and water balances in the blood, but nephritis interferes with this function, often causing the bloodstream to become overloaded with excess elements such as water and salt. The body's ability to utilize protein is also often impaired during kidney infection, and protein, or albumin can be abnormally excreted in the urine.

Symptoms of nephritis are chills, fever, urgent and frequent urination, back and abdominal pain, loss of appetite, nausea and vomiting. Blood in the urine and cloudy urine are also symptoms.

This study revealed that urine injections significantly reduced the symptoms and successfully eliminated kidney infections in most cases:

"The modern therapeutic tendency for acute infectious diseases is typically an etiologic tendency; it is exactly from this basis that the concept of vaccine therapy, for example, autogenous (individual, natural) vaccines and protein-therapy, has entered today's standard practice. Actually, there are many infectious diseases for which this type of treatment is utilized...

Since 1926, Professor Silvestrini has been using urine vaccine autotherapy for cases of nephritis; however until now, a systematic and particularly a clinically statistical study which could offer a precise indication of its effectiveness had not been compiled. Therefore, I have collected the medical histories of numerous patients who underwent this therapy during previous years, and, in addition, a group of others which I was able to personally follow and administer laboratory investigations with the goal of obtaining as many clinical observations as was possible.

CASE STUDIES

CASE III.   A patient came into the clinic presenting albuminuria (protein) and blood cells [in the urine], fever, edema (water retention, or swelling), and cyanosis (blue discoloration of the skin). The patient was treated with a course of seven injections (7 cc. each) of auto-urine vaccine. An examination of the patient's urine was done after the third injection and showed only small traces of albumin and blood cells and the edema and cyanosis had disappeared. After completing the treatment course, the patient was discharged from the hospital, completely healed.

CASE IV.   The patient came into the clinic presenting albuminuria and blood cells in the urine, temperature, but no edema. The patient received urine injections, and after the eighth injection, all of his symptoms had gone into total remission. Three weeks after the treatments, the patient continues to remain completely healed.

CASE V.   Upon entering the clinic, the patient's examination revealed considerable protein and blood in the urine and visual disturbances in the left eye. After only three injections of the urine vaccine, the symptoms completely disappeared and the patient was released completely cured.

This Italian research study on nephritis and urine therapy was an extremely in-depth report, detailing 18 cases of clinical nephritis which were successfully treated with urine injections.

Another similar study on the treatment of nephritis, entitled, Treatment Of Glomer-ulonephritis By Antigen, published in the London Lancet, in Dec., 1936, by Dr. H.B. Day, (London), also demonstrated the effectiveness of a simple, natural urine extract on several cases of both acute and chronic nephritis:

> *"Treatment by injection of urine extract appeared of distinct value in acute glomerulonephritis and for exacerbations or relapses in chronic active forms of the disease...In chronic cases, the effect of this treatment is often striking."*

Day also noted that:

> *Tests on patients without nephritis showed that the urine extract, even in large doses, had no adverse effect on renal function or on the blood pressure.*

TITLE: *TREATMENT OF COLIBACILLARY CYSTITIS WITH AUTO-URINE THERAPY,* 1935, by Dr. M. Garotescu, published in the medical journal, Romania Medicala.

Report #7

In this report, the author, Dr. Garotescu, describes his experiences in treating cystitis, a painful inflammation, or infection of the bladder which commonly affects women and can lead to more serious conditions, such as kidney infections.

Dr. Garotescu treated numerous cases of cystitis with injections of the patients' own urine, and discovered that these treatments produced excellent results, which were corroborated by laboratory tests showing that the cystitis bacteria had completely disappeared after the urine injection treatments. For example:

CASE #1: A thirty-two year-old woman with typical symptoms of cystitis including frequent, painful urination; also complained of chronic constipation for which she has been taking laxatives unsuccessfully for several years. She was treated with 12 urine injections and all symptoms completely disappeared. The success of the treatment was verified by laboratory tests which showed a complete absence of colibaccilli (cystitis bacteria) in her urine.

CASE #2: A 28 year-old woman complaining of frequent and painful urination. Laboratory analysis of urine sample revealed the presence of numerous colonies of colibacilli. Patient was given 4 injections of auto-urine, after which all symptoms and signs of the infection were completely ameliorated.

Dr. Garotescu reported that he gave 220 urine injections to patients without any adverse side effects whatever, other than an occasional, temporary redness and swelling at the site of the injection which is commonly reported with urine injections, or injections of any kind.

Report #8

TITLE: *VIRUCIDAL (RABIES AND POLIOMYELITIS) ACTIVITY OF AQUEOUS UREA SOLUTIONS,* 1936, by Dr. Eaton M. MacKay and Dr. Charles R. Schroeder, published for the American Proceedings of the Society of Experimental Biology.

SUBJECT: *DESTRUCTION OF THE RABIES AND POLIO VIRUS BY UREA.*

This report on urea's ability to destroy viruses is extremely interesting and important in view of the fact that even today, almost 60 years after this study was published, there is still no medical cure or effective drug treatment for viral infections. And as we know, viruses can be deadly.

After experimenting with the effect of urea on the polio and rabies viruses, McKay and Schroeder report that:

> *"...The effect of urea in strong concentration on these viruses (rabies and polio) proved interesting. As first recorded by Spiro and Ramsden,* **urea in aqueous solution has a remarkable ability to 'dissolve' proteins...**
>
> *We conclude...that the strong solution of urea not only attenuates (weakens) or dilutes the poliomyelitis virus in the sense that it is non-infective but* **actually destroys it...**
>
> **Urea is such a relatively inactive substance and certainly not a protoplasmic poison such as are most virucidal agents that it is in a way surprising that rabies and poliomyelitis are killed so easily by urea solutions...**
>
> *It is true that neutral and inactive as it is, urea, like alkalies, denatures protein when dissolving it and this reaction may be associated with the death of the virus. This denaturation occurs in a very few minutes..."*

This report appears to hold important implications for the treatment of the AIDS virus, HIV. Because concentrated urea has been proven to destroy viruses without harming the body, oral urine therapy, which increases urea concentrations (see Dr. D. Kaye), would logically be an extremely important addition to treatment regimens; especially in view of the fact that urine therapy also provides a wide variety of antibodies (including HIV antibodies in infected patients) and other important immune defense supporting agents.

No one with HIV or AIDS can afford to ignore the information on urine therapy, especially considering the danger and ineffectiveness of the 'accepted' AIDS treatments such as AZT. A separate section on AIDS and urine therapy is presented further on in this chapter. Again, because urine therapy is easily accessed, inexpensive and proven to be completely safe, there is absolutely no downside risk to using it in treating AIDS and other viral iinfections.

TITLE: *TREATMENT OF INFECTED WOUNDS WITH UREA,* 1938, by Leon Muldavis (Senior Casualty Officer at the Royal Free Hospital, London) and Jean M. Holtzman (Demonstrator in Physiology, London School of Medicine for Women). Published in the English medical journal, The London Lancet.

Report #9

SUBJECT: *HEALING INFECTED WOUNDS, SKIN ULCERS AND BURNS WITH UREA*

Drawing on earlier research into the treatment of wounds with urea, Muldavis and Holtzman began using urea crystals extensively in their hospital treatments of serious wounds and burns:

> *"The protein solvent properties of urea were first investigated by Spiro (1900) and independently by Ramsden (1902)... Symmers and Kirk (1915) reported on its bactericidal properties together with its use in the treatment of wounds. In spite of this article, the use of urea for wound therapy has apparently enjoyed little popularity in this country [England].*
>
> *In America, however, it has recently been used for the treatment of various infected wounds by Robinson (1936) and by Holder and McKay (1937), who found it extremely efficient. Moreover, it is a substance that is readily obtainable in quantity and is both cheap and stable. For these reasons it was thought desirable to test its efficacy in the casualty department of the Royal Free Hospital (London)...*
>
> *No toxic effects have been recorded even though the urea has been applied in solid form. We therefore decided to use both the saturated solution and crystals throughout.*
>
> *The procedure employed was as follows: The wounds were syringed free from pus and necrotic (dead) material with a saturated solution of urea, excessive moisture was removed and the urea crystals were then liberally applied. Waxed paper was placed next to the crystals to keep*

them in contact with the wound and to prevent the dressing becoming soaked.

For a period of six months cases of the following types have been treated: (1) Abscesses – superficial and deep lesions, (2) Infected traumatic wounds of all descriptions, (3) infected hematomas (bruised areas), (4) Cellulitis, (inflamed subcutaneous tissue), (5) Septic wounds due to burns of 2nd, 3rd, and 4th degree, (6) varicose ulcers, (7) carbuncles (external staph infections), (8) Infected tenosynovitis (inflamed tendons) of the hand. In all, 170 cases have been treated. Notes were kept on the progress of all of them...

With a view to comparing the efficiency of urea with that of other solutions, the cases at first selected for treatment were those which had either behaved sluggishly with other antiseptics or had actually retrogressed. The results obtained were so favorable that we began to use urea more generally.

TYPICAL CASES

CASE 1.   A man aged 27 presented a varicose ulcer...of the left leg...He had it for nearly 18 months without its having healed. During this time it had been treated with Eastoplast and various other substances. At the time the urea treatment was begun the ulcer was of oval irregular outline with everted swollen edges and a floor covered with a whitish, foul smelling slough. The ulcer received the urea dressings daily for 14 days. After 2 days the foul odor had disappeared and after 4 days the base of the ulcer was covered by a mass of bright red granulations (new tissue). By the 14th day the skin edges had grown in and the size of the ulcer was 3/4 by 1/2 in. The floor was dry. The patient had a dry dressing and was discharged. The ulcer was again examined 10 days after the patient's discharge and was found to be completely healed.

CASE 2.   A male aged 47 had a septic area on the...third right finger. This was drained but discharge of pus continued. The wound was opened again when it was found that the infection had entered the tendon sheath. Adequate drainage was provided and the finger X-rayed. The wound was then treated with eusol baths. After several days there was no attempt at healing. Urea treatment was started and after 3 days the slough was removed thus exposing the underlying tendon. Healthy granulations (new tissue) were present at this time. The urea treatment was continued. The patient was discharged 22 days after the treatment was begun, the wound having healed completely. There was no loss of function...

As will be seen from the above, we have used urea in a variety of casualty department cases. Owing to the extreme diffusibility of urea even the deepest wound can be treated effectively.

A very definite response to urea treatment is nearly always obtained after two or three applications...septic burns, even though they cover a very wide area, under this treatment become clean and form granulations so quickly that the surrounding epithelium is able to grow in with but little delay. The same prompt response is often obtained in varicose ulcers. Coupled with this is a considerable decrease of edema as the local circulatory conditions improve. For the carbuncles (external staph infections), treated, we found urea preferable to any other dressing after initial incision...

In none of the cases of our series did we observe any skin reaction which could be called a urea dermatitis (rash), nor have we evidence of any toxic effects. We never saw a spread of sepsis (infection) under urea treatment or any undermining of the wound edges.

The advantages of the urea treatment are as follows: (1) It is cheap, the crystals costing one shilling per pound...(2) It produces no dermatitis. (3) It deodorizes foul smelling wounds. (4) By dissolving necrotic (dead) material, it produces a clean wound, so allowing healing to proceed. (5) Local circulatory conditions are improved and healthy granulations (new tissues) are produced. (6) It has no toxic effect and causes no necrosis (death) of living material. For this reason, unlike strong anti-septics it does not destroy the "leucocytic barrier" essential to the organism's defense. (7) Urea treatment has been successful where other treatments have failed. (8) We found no contra-indications to its use."

It seems extremely unfortunate, after reading this study, that safe, effective and inexpensive urea was ignored as a general antiseptic and wound treatment in favor of cortisone and antibiotic creams. Cortisone has been proven to be dangerous and toxic and antibiotics destroy good bacteria along with the bad. Also by using antibiotics routinely, we have greatly reduced their effectiveness as bacterial strains have developed increasing resistance to them.

Report #10

TITLE: *THE EFFECT OF URINE EXTRACTS ON PEPTIC ULCER,* 1941, by David J. Sandweiss, M.D., M.H. Sugarman, M.D., M.H.F. Friedman, Ph.D., H.C. Saltzstein, M.D., (Research aided by grants from the Mendelson Fund and Parke-Davis & Co.).

SUBJECT: *TREATMENT OF STOMACH ULCERS WITH URINE EXTRACTS*

This is a report on clinical and laboratory studies indicating that urine extracts taken from pregnancy urine and normal urine, when given intravenously or injected, have beneficial and therapeutic effects on chronic duodenal ulcers and other types of stomach ulcers in humans and on experimentally induced animal stomach ulcers.

The researchers reported, among other things, that:

1) urine contains a type of gastric secretory suppressant (or antacid) called urogastrone, that can protect against irritation of the stomach lining that may lead to ulcers.

2) certain urine extracts also encouraged healing of ulcers by stimulating the growth of new cells, tissues and blood vessels in the damaged area.

The study also discusses a pregnancy urine extract called Antuitrin S which was reported to have a beneficial therapeutic effect on experimentally induced ulcers in animals..

In the report, urine extract therapy is compared to other ulcer drug treatments and diet changes and it was found in human testing that:

> *"...a higher per cent of those [ulcer patients] treated with urine extract became symptom free during treatment (thus, a greater number enjoyed a maintenance diet sooner) and a much higher percent enjoyed longer symptom free intervals (thus, a greater number continued with a more liberal diet over a much longer period of time).*

This study references 13 other research studies before 1941 that were also conducted on the beneficial effects of urine extracts in the treatment of stomach ulcers.

TITLE: *THE WATER OF LIFE*, (book) 1944, by John Armstrong.   *Report #11*

This book was not written by a doctor or researcher, but it's the most compelling and powerful book of testimonials ever written on the use of urine therapy and deserves to be included in any work on urine therapy.

John Armstrong was just an "ordinary" Englishman with an extraordinary insight. When he contracted tuberculosis at the age of 34 and later diabetes, he went to various doctors for help, but after two years of unsuccessful treatments, decided to look for his own solution to his health problems. The solution he discovered was urine therapy.

After fasting for forty-five days on nothing but urine and water Armstrong reported that:

> "I felt and was 'an entirely new man'. I weighed 140 lbs., was full of vim and looked about eleven years younger than I actually was."

Armstrong was so amazed at his own recovery, that he began to advise other people on how to cure themselves with urine fasting. His technique was so successful that many hundreds of people with everything from cancer to heart disease, gangrene, kidney disease, venereal disease, obesity, prostrate problems and many other difficult disorders came to Armstrong for help and were cured. Armstrong himself reportedly lived healthily and happily ever after, well into his eighties, by maintaining a good diet, a healthful lifestyle and by ingesting a small daily dose of urine.

One thing lacking in Armstrong's book is scientific evidence, but the stories are so full of the incredible drama of dreadfully sick people getting miraculously well that most people who read it cease to care about corroborative laboratory studies.

Armstrong's book is a wonderful inspiration, but the fact that so much scientific evidence supporting urine therapy does exist needs be recognized and made public because until it is, the majority of people will be scared away from urine therapy by doctors and medical practitioners who insist that there are no laboratory and clinical studies supporting it.

Also, Armstrong's method of extended urine and water fasts is very radical and is definitely not advisable for home use, especially since Armstrong supervised his patients extremely carefully and provided certain conditions for his fasts which are not easily duplicated today. John Arm-strong's book is an inspiring compilation of testimonials and makes excellent reading for everyone interested in urine therapy.

Report #12   **TITLE:** *THE ACTION OF UREA AND SOME OF ITS DERIVATIVES ON BACTERIA,* by Louis Weinstein and Alice McDonald, 1946, From the Evans Memorial, Massachusetts Memorial Hospitals, and the Department of Medicine, Boston,Massachusetts.

SUBJECT: THE BACTERIA-DESTROYING PROPERTIES OF UREA

DISCUSSION: THE POTENTIAL DANGER OF USING SYNTHETIC URINE DERIVATIVES.

This study is only one of several conducted on the anti-bacterial prop-erties of urea by the two researchers, Weinstein and McDonald. In this report, they discuss previous research into the antibacterial effect of urea and report that their studies also confirmed that urea will both inhibit the growth and destroy many different types of bacteria such as those that cause dysentery, typhoid, and staph and strep infections:

> *"Urea and urethane are bacteriostatic and bactericidal for a number of gram-negative and gram-positive bacteria..."*

In other words, this study proved, as did others like it, that urea can stop the growth or kill many different types of disease bacteria.

This particular study on urea is also good example of why synthetic drug compounds should not routinely be considered for use in the place of basic or natural medicinal elements.

As Weinstein and McDonald stated, they used both urea and a chemi-cally synthesized urea compound called urethane to kill bacteria and they recommended both urea and urethane for medical use as anti-bac-terial agents.

Weinstein and McDonald discovered that urethane (made by heating urea and mixing it with alcohol and other synthetic agents) was sometimes a faster and deadlier "kill" than urea alone on bacteria, and so emphasized its use over simple urea. But what they didn't realize at the time was that urethane has a carcinogenic (cancer-causing) effect on the body.

As the **Fourth Annual Report on Carcinogens,** 1985 stated: *"This substance [urethane] may reasonably be anticipated to be a carcinogen"*. A review of urethane's carcinogenic action was also reported in the journal of Advanced Cancer Research in 1968.

So you can see how extremely dangerous errors can be made by scientists experimenting with new and "improved" synthetic drugs. In Weinstein and McDonald's day, there was no way of knowing or predicting how urethane would affect the body in the long term. And the same is true today of new drugs that initially seem like miracle cures but later turn out to be deadly substances.

Compound urine-derivative drugs may seem superior in the minds of medical researchers, and even consumers, but what good are they if they later prove to be harmful or even fatal? Simple urea and urine have been shown to be safe over nearly a full century of scientific study and use, so it certainly makes sense to start using them routinely in medicine before resorting to potentially dangerous compound chemical drugs.

TITLE: *URINE THERAPY,* 1947, by Professor J. Plesch, M.D., From an article in the English medical journal, *The Medical Press* (London).

Report #13

SUBJECT: USE OF URINE THERAPY IN THE TREATMENT OF INFECTIOUS DISEASES, ASTHMA, ALLERGIES, MIGRAINES, VIRAL INFECTIONS, HAYFEVER, DIABETES, GOUT, DYSFUNCTION OF THE ADRENAL AND THYROID GLANDS, HEART CONDITIONS.

Dr. Plesch, an English physician, used natural urine injections in his medical practice extensively and with excellent success on a large variety of disease conditions:

> *"...In fact, my recommendation to use the urine of the infected person for auto-vaccination is only an extension of the methods of Jenner and Pasteur and therefore it is strange that auto-urine vaccination has not*

been used before. **The main difference between the Pasteur-Jenner methods and auto-urine therapy lies in the fact that by inoculating the fresh urine of the patient the active infectious material has been weakened by passage through the recipient's own body.**

I am convinced from my experience that it is worthwhile investigating this method systematically with respect to all infectious diseases, including poliomyelitis, etc.

Moreover, during the application of this therapy, I observed some remarkable effects. Among my first patients whom I treated by urine therapy was a typical case of **asthma.** *Immediately after the first injection and before the vaccination effect had time to develop, this patient lost his daily attacks of asthma.*

Following up this clue, I found that anaphylactic (allergic) persons could be desensitized by the auto-urine injection. Subsequent investigation convinced me that auto-urine therapy could be used with considerable advantage against all kinds of anaphylactic **(allergic) diseases, such as hayfever, urticaria, (hives), disfunction of the intestinal tract such as cramps, etc. It also relieved migraine and other spastic conditions.**

Since I started the auto-urine therapy three years ago, I have given several hundred injections and I have not come across a single case where the patient suffered any harm.

It is for this reason, and because the method is so simple that is can be used by any practitioner without any difficulties, that I decided to publish my findings at this early stage.

The observations which I have quoted are without doubt sufficient to indicate to the expert that a completely new field of research is being opened up which may entail considerable additions to our knowledge of bacteriology, immunology and serology.

The fresh urine of men is practically sterile and that of women, too, if the exterior genitalia have been cleaned previously. For purposes of immediate injection the urine may therefore be collected directly into sterile vessels...

The application is very simple indeed. The most suitable method is intragluteal injection. When using urine as an auto-vaccine I found that usually one injection of a quarter to a half cc. of fresh urine is sufficient. In anaphylactic (allergy) cases I have found it useful to start with 5 cc. of fresh urine and to repeat the injections with diminishing doses down to 1/2 cc. of fresh urine...

Thus urine can be used for immunization or desensitization. Treatment **with the patient's own urine is indicated against bacterial or virus infections and against allergic conditions...Moreover, the hormonal end products and enzymes contained in the urine make it probable that this method may be useful against metabolic disturbances such as diabetes and gout and against derangements of the ovarial or thyroid, etc. functions."**

CASE STUDIES

JAUNDICE
(1) Miss M. – 14 years old. At school several attacks of icterus (jaundice). Since 2/1/45 depressed, headaches, no appetite, coated tongue, somewhat increased temperature. Blown up feeling in the abdomen, pains in the right hypogastrium. 13/1, Fully developed jaundice, urine dark brown. 16/1, Intragluteal injection of 1/2 cc. own urine. No local reaction. 31/1. Jaundice symptoms in the skin, sclera and urine disappeared entirely. Feeling well again.

ULCERS, DIGESTIVE PROBLEMS
(2) Lance-Corporal L. – 28 years of age. Joined New Zealand forces 1942. Contracted infective hepatitis in Africa. After hospital treatment the icterus (jaundice) disappeared, a feeling of weakness, intestinal troubles and depression remained. In the following years repeated hospital treatment. Has been X-rayed several times for duodenal ulcer and gallstones. Since then he dragged himself about complaining of loss of appetite, tiredness and indifference, pains in the abdomen after food, constipation, distension and abdominal discomfort with flatulence. 14/3/45, Injection with 1/2 cc. fresh urine.

The patient's report is as follows – felt better after injection. 15/3, felt normal, bowels regular. 16/3, Feeling quite normal except for tenderness in stomach. 17/3, No change. 21/3, Quite well, but tenderness in stomach worse. 24/3, Sore throat, feverish, feeling weak and depressed. 25/3, Cannot eat, sore throat, feverish, weak. 26/3, Eating. Sore throat better. 29/3, Feels quite well, bowels regular, strength returned...3/4, No change, still in high spirits, feel well. 26/8, Patient writes: I enjoyed 100 percent improvement in my health, I am eating well, sleeping well and feel very active with no stomach tenderness or sickness.

ASTHMA
(4) Mister T. – 17 years of age. First asthma attack at the age of one:- – "Flushy, cyanotic, gasping for breath. Attacks last for hours." Change of domicile brought no relief. Daily attacks. Asthmatic deformation of thorax. 12/10/45, Injection of 2 cc. fresh urine. No asthma until 8/11/45, after exertion. In the afternoon 2 cc. of fresh urine. Within five minutes attack ceases. Strong local reaction for 30 hours. 30/12, Starting cold, but with only very slight attacks of asthma. Since last injection no strong attack. 12/4/46. After renewed injection on 25/4 oí 1/2 cc. of fresh urine, the attacks stop.

HAYFEVER
(5) Mr. J.B. – 44 years of age. Since childhood severe hayfever at the end of May. 31/5/46, 2 cc. fresh urine injected. 8/6, new injection of 2 cc. 9/6, slight running and burning sensation of the eyes began but the hayfever did not develop further and disappeared entirely on 20/6/46.

MIGRAINES, MENSTRUAL PROBLEMS
(8) Lady H. – 32 years of age. Married. Complaints since childhood. Complaints about distention, flatulence, digestive troubles...attacks of severe migraine (which) occur regularly before menstruation. 4/4/45, 2 cc. of fresh urine injected. Injection repeated on 10/4 and 17/4. In the last two years no digestive troubles, no migraine attacks any more before menstruation. Other spastic symptoms have also disappeared.

ARTHRITIS, HEART PROBLEMS
(9) Mr. F. – 43 years. At 20 years of age polyarthritis with chorea (nervous disorder). Mitral insufficiency which led to an enormous dilation of the left auricle. Severe attacks of heart weakness. In the last four years repeated fits of pulmonal edema with bloody sputum. For the last two years this condition is aggravated by bronchial asthma. First injection 12/1/46 with 3 cc. fresh urine. On the day

of injection patient feels much better, after 24 hours severe attack of asthma. Heart becomes weak and must be treated. Only slight asthma; on 3/3 2 cc. fresh urine injected.

Severe attack of heart weakness, sleep is disturbed. Since then patient recovered; not only have his attacks of bronchial asthma ceased, but the condition of the heart has also improved substantially. He is able to lie down again and can take some exercise. Since the last injection patient does not require any cardiac medicine.

WHOOPING COUGH

(3) Master W. – 4-1/2 years of age. Developed a severe fit of coughing with vomiting. Whooping-cough epidemic in the village. Urine injection given...In the night, severe fit of coughing with thick phlegm and mucus, sick feeling...Next day, feeling much better in every way, no whooping or return of chronic asthma. His mother later writes "Child better than ever, is free from asthma since the first injections [several weeks ago]", Have seen the child [four months after injections]. He is developing physically without any disturbance. Chronic eczema and blepharedenitis (inflammation of the eyelids) also healed.

Plesch reports on many more successful cases during his clinical use of urine therapy and the results are so impressive that it seems hard to believe that urine therapy has received so little public attention as an over-all medical treatment for both adults and children.

TITLE: *ON THE EFFECT OF HUMAN URINE ON TUBERCULE BACILLI,* 1951 by Dr. K.B. Bjornesjo, From the Department of Medical Chemistry, Uppsala, Sweden.

Report #14

SUBJECT: ANTI-TUBERCULE EFFECT OF URINE

Although some medical researchers for many years had been aware that different body fluids such as serum and saliva had an inhibitory effect on tuberculosis bacteria, Bjornesjo, a Scandinavian researcher, discovered that urine was much more effective that any other body fluids in arresting the growth of tuberculosis bacilli:

"In a preliminary experiment performed in this laboratory employing (solutions of) saliva, serum and urine from different subjects...it became apparent that under the experimental conditions the inhibitory effect of saliva and serum was very weak...On the other hand urine seemed to have a considerably stronger inhibitory effect and a concentration of 50 per cent urine in (a) medium completely inhibited the growth of the tubercule bacilli in most cases..."

Bjornesjo conducted extensive testing of the anti-tuberculosis property of urine and concluded that:

1) The majority of urines examined showed a strong inhibitory effect of the growth of the tubercule bacteria.

2) Human urine also has a bactericidal (bacteria-killing) effect on tuberculosis bacteria.

3) The anti-TB element of urine was shown in laboratory tests to be present in tuberculin positive and negative individuals and also in healthy vegetarians and in patients with active tuberculosis.

4) The presence of urine in the urinary tract exerts an anti-TB effect that can influence the course and spreading of tuberculosis in the urinary tract itself.

Bjornesjo's experiments clearly demonstrated that human urine could inhibit the growth and even completely destroy the tuberculosis bacteria, but he was unable to identify which element in urine is responsible for its anti-tubercule activity.

Actually, Bjornesjo tried for many years to determine the anti-tubercular element in urine, so that it could be isolated, but he was never successful. It wasn't until 1965 that Japanese researchers discovered and isolated this mystery anti-TB element in urine – 14 years after Bjornesjo's first attempts.

Bjornesjo considered the possibility that urea is the antitubercular agent in urine, but he ruled this out, perhaps prematurely. In his experiments, Bjornesjo only considered the anti-bacterial strength of a 2 per cent solution of urea, which is the average amount of urea found in normal urine. However, as later research in 1961 (see Dr. Schlegel), showed, urea in higher concentrations (8%) does inhibit or destroy both gram negative and gram positive bacteria. So even though specific anti-tubercular agents other than urea are in urine, urea most likely also plays a role.

But again, if we were to use a urea extract alone in treating TB, rather than whole urine, the important anti-tubercular element in whole urine that Bjornesjo discovered would be eliminated from our treatment, which indicates that a combination of whole urine and urea could offer an extremely effective TB treatment.

TITLE: *STUDIES ON THE TUBER-CULOINHIBITORY PROPER-TIES OF ASCORBIC ACID DERIVATIVES AND THEIR POSSIBLE ROLE IN INHIBITION OF TUBERCULE BACILLI BY URINE*, 1954, by Dr. Quentin Myrvik, R. Weiser, B. Houglum, and L. Berger. From the Department of Microbiology, University of Washington School of Medicine, Seattle, Washington.

Report #15

When Bjornesjo discovered that urine can inhibit or destroy the bacteria that causes tuberculosis, rather than use this information to support traditional urine therapy, he conducted several more intensive research studies in an attempt to determine what exactly it was in the urine that killed the TB bacillus so that it could be isolated and produced in drug form but, as we said his research was unsuccessful.

This particular study was another attempt by several other researchers to find the mystery element in urine that destroyed TB bacteria and they suggested that it might be the ascorbic acid (vitamin C) in urine:

> "The idea that the ascorbic acid of urine and serum may exert tuber-culostatic action is not new...These observations are not inconsistent with the concept of the present writers that the tuberculostatic activity of urine reported by Bjornesjo in some way depends on ascorbic acid."

This assumption was incorrect. It wasn't until several years later, in the following study done in 1965, that Japanese researchers were able to partially identify what it was in urine that stopped the growth of TB bacteria.

Report #16 **TITLE:** *ISOLATION FROM HUMAN URINE OF A POLYPEPTIDE HAVING MARKED TUBERCULOSTATIC ACTIVITY,* 1965, by Shusuke Tsuji, et. al., From the Fifth Division of the Tuberculosis Research Institute, Kyoto University, Japan.

In one of the opening statements of this report, the researchers comment that: *"The vast majority of Japanese adults are tuberculin positive..."* which is apparently why the laboratory evidence of urine's anti-TB property was of interest to Japanese researchers and why they conducted their own search for the anti-TB element in urine:

> *"In short, although it has been a well known fact that human urine has definite capacity to inhibit the growth of tubercule bacilli...the chemical nature of the active substance has been obscure. In our investigations it has become clear that at least one of the active agents is a polypeptide."*

Although these researchers did identify one of the active elements in urine's tuberculostatic activity as a polypeptide (which is a chain of amino acids), they also admitted that there are other "as yet undetermined agents" responsible for urine's anti-TB property.

Most of us in the U.S. have no concept of the seriousness of tuberculosis, because our plentiful food sources, excellent sanitation and modern drugs seemed to have eliminated this formerly dreaded disease. But only recently, this article, which was mentioned in Chapter 3, revealed that TB is a modern-day threat:

The Associated Press
Friday, October 8, 1993

> *WASHINGTON – New cases of tuberculosis are increasing at an alarming rate, posing a special threat to the poor and people with the virus that causes acquired immune deficiency syndrome (AIDS), congressional analysts reported Thursday...The congressional report said EFFORTS TO COMBAT TUBERCULOSIS ARE COMPLICATED BECAUSE OF THE EMERGENCE OF STRAINS RESISTANT TO ANTI-TB DRUGS... (my caps)*

The fact that TB and other disease microorganisms are now resistant to many of our chemical drugs should set off an alarm somewhere in our consciousness. The whole point of evolution is adaptation and survival, and as this article, and others like it reveal, disease germs are obviously surviving by adapting natural defenses to our chemical drugs – but are we adapting natural defenses to the germs?

How can our natural immune defenses possibly develop and adapt normally to new and stronger strains of disease microorganisms, when we constantly override our bodies' natural responses to disease with unnatural drugs? For years, we've interfered with even the most basic of our bodies' natural defenses, such as fever, by substituting chemical drugs for critical natural immune responses to infections and disease.

A crucial fact that we have overlooked in this era of modern medicine is that the body itself has the innate natural ability to adapt and change to new disease influences, but chemical drugs do not.

We might think that medical scientists can keep coming up with newer and stronger drugs to combat new microorganisms, but drug research isn't routinely successful and it takes many years to develop new treatments. Many of us could well be victims of these new bacteria and viruses, such as AIDS, long before our scientists figure out what these organisms are and how they kill us.

Natural medicinal substances, like herbs or urine, or homeopathic medicines, are traditionally known for their ability to gently assist and support our bodies' own immune functions rather than overriding them through strong chemical intervention, which is why we need to emphasize their use and decrease our dependence on drugs. The 'immune-bashing' methods of today's conventional medicine may prove to be our undoing if we continue to use them as irresponsibly as we do today.

TITLE: *EFFECT OF UREA ON CEREBROSPINAL FLUID PRESSURE IN HUMAN SUBJECTS*, 1956, From the Journal of the American Medical Association.   *Report #17*

SUBJECT: REDUCTION OF CEREBROSPINAL FLUID PRESSURE WITH UREA; USE OF UREA AS A DIURETIC AND IN MENINGITIS.

This is an interesting and precedent-setting study. The two university doctors who conducted this research were intrigued by the possibility that urea, which was known to be an excellent natural diuretic, could also be used to reduce excess fluid pressure on the brain and spinal cord which were created by various disease conditions or abnormalities such as brain tumors, hydrocephalus (water on the brain), cerebral hemorrhage or meningitis.

Excessive intracranial pressure can be extremely dangerous and, if severe and unrelieved, can cause death, so it is of utmost importance to relieve this pressure or inflammation as quickly and effectively as possible without causing harmful side effects. Swelling and pressure in the cerebral cavity and spinal area also create problems during brain surgery.

The researchers, in this preliminary study, laid the groundwork for the use of urea in reducing such pressure:

> *"The purpose of this report is to describe findings in a preliminary study to determine the safety and efficiency with which urea might be used intravenously for the purpose of reducing intracranial pressure. Many (other) agents have been used for this purpose but each has some undesirable action that limits or prohibits its use."*

In the study, the doctors report good results in clinical trials on patients with excessive cranial pressure:

> *"...it was found that the average pressure drop produced by urea was 4.5 times greater than that caused by sucrose or dextrose (and)...the urea effects were much longer lasting."*

The clinical use of urea as a diuretic is also discussed:

> *"Urea has, however, been used clinically for other purposes than reduction of intracranial tension. It has long been recognized to be an effective diuretic agent. Salter states: 'One of the most effective diuretic agents is urea, nature's own non-electrolytic diuretic.' For the purpose of promoting diuresis it is administered by the oral route, 20 gm. two to five times daily."*

Urea's successful historical use in combination with sulfa drugs is also commented on in relation to treating meningitis with urea:

> *"LaLonde and Gardner gave urea in conjunction with sulfonamides in the treatment of meningitis...*
>
> *It is thus evident that the clinical use of urea is not without precedent. It is a normal body metabolite that is well tolerated in large doses..."*

The success of this preliminary study on the use of urea in neurosurgery encouraged further research. The next study was one of several follow-up research projects and clinical trials that established urea as an effective agent in treating many different disorders involving excessive fluid pressure in the body.

TITLE: *UREA – NEW USE OF AN OLD AGENT,* 1957. From a Symposium on Surgery of the Head and Neck.

Report #18

SUBJECT: UREA TREATMENT OF EXCESS CEREBRAL AND SPINAL PRESSURE, INOPERABLE BRAIN TUMORS, EDEMA (FLUID PRESSURE) OF THE BRAIN, PREMENSTRUAL WATER RETENTION, MENINGITIS, CHRONIC GLAUCOMA, HYDRO-CEPHALUS, DELIRIUM TREMENS AND EPILEPSY

Because of the encouraging results of the previous urea research, doctors conducted this more intensive study which included extensive clinical trials using urea on 300 patients with a wide variety of disorders including brain tumors, hydrocephalus (water on the brain), migraines, glaucoma, meningitis, brain abscess, retinal detachment and premenstrual edema.

Results of these trials were so successful, doctors concluded that:

> *"This agent (urea) has a definite place in the therapeutic armamentarium of neurologists and neurosurgeons... The combination of urea and 10 per cent invert sugar is now used routinely in the neurosurgical service for intravenous administration..."*

There were reports on remarkable cases in which the clinical use of urea was literally life-saving as in the case of a woman who developed severe swelling or edema of the brain after the surgical removal of a small brain tumor:

> *"...On the fourth postoperative day, she developed signs of increased intracranial pressure. In the course of a few hours, she became progressively lethargic and then suddenly she became unresponsive...Her pupils became dilated and fixed, her systolic blood pressure rose... Preparations were underway to take her to the operating room for the removal of a bone flap.*
>
> *Urea was administered intravenously as an emergency measure. Within 20 minutes from the start of injection her blood pressure had*

returned to normal and her pupils began to react...to light. From this time on, her recovery was uneventful...

In this case, urea was definitely life-saving, because prior to its administration the patient was in critical condition and her survival until surgical decompression could be done was unlikely...

In many similar instances urea was found to be life-saving."

The researchers commented on the urea treatment of another patient who had a brain tumor surgically removed but developed another massive brain tumor three months later:

"...the patient received 256 ml. of 30 per cent urea. The bulging mass had completely disappeared by the end of two hours..."

On the diuretic properties of urea, the doctors reported:

"Urea is one of the most useful nonmetabolized, nonelectrolyte diuretics. Its diuretic property does not diminish after prolonged administration, as is the case with acid-producing salts."

In observing its effect on relieving fluid pressure on the eyes in glaucoma and other ophthalmic patients, researchers stated that:

"Urea has been administered to 25 patients with acute and chronic glaucoma, orbital tumors, retinal detachment and other conditions. In comparing the effect of urea with [Diamox] on intraocular pressure, urea was found to be more effective..."

Urea, as studies and doctors and researchers have proven, is a safe, non-toxic, remarkably effective and inexpensive diuretic – but unfortunately, it's not even listed in any diuretic capacity in the Physician's Desk Reference (PDR) which is the doctors guide to approved drug treatments.

But Diamox, the synthetic diuretic which doctors said was less effective than urea, is listed in the PDR – even though it's been proven that urea was safer and more effective than Diamox and several other synthetic diuretics and urea is FDA approved. So why should Diamox be recommended to physicians rather than urea for diuretic use?

Diamox is a sulfa drug and like all sulfa drugs, it can be dangerous. *The Physician's Desk Reference* (1992) warns that "fatalities have occurred" with Diamox and that it can cause severe allergic reactions, bone marrow depression, a decrease in white blood cells, anemia, and a host of other equally horrific side effects.

On the other hand, urea is an effective, inexpensive diuretic and has no side-effects or toxicity and it's FDA approved. But doctors don't know this – instead they are directed to prescribe Diamox or some other 'recommended' form of diuretic drug treatment being pushed by the drug companies. It's hard to believe that the conventional medical establishment is complaining to patients and the media about "snake-oil" sellers and phony medical claims that the public supposedly needs protection from, when obviously cogent medical research like that done on urea is so completely ignored.

Another point to consider is that synthetic diuretics alter the sodium/potassium (or electrolyte) balance of the body which can cause havoc with your health. But as the researchers pointed out, urea is a non-electrolytic diuretic that safely reduces fluid pressure in the body and its effects last longer than other diuretics.

Most people and practicing doctors have never heard of the oral use of urea, but it's not uncommon in medical research. The doctors in this study and many other researchers have given large doses of urea by mouth, as well as intravenously:

> *"...Urea has also been used by mouth in tablet form, or in powder dissolved in such [things] as unsweetened fruit juices..."*

This study like so many before it, again proved that urea was a safe medicinal agent, even in large doses, as well as being extremely simple and effective:

> Dosages. *"...After urea was proved to be a safe agent which was well tolerated in large doses, the dosage was increased until, today, in the majority of the patients, it is 1 gram per kilogram of body weight..."*

Because of the success of the preliminary clinical trials using urea on a variety of disease conditions doctors recommended that:

> *"Further trials of urea are warranted in [the treatment of]: encephalopathies (abnormal conditions of the structure of function of tissues of the brain)... Meniere's disease (disease of the inner ear), 'premenstrual edema', eclampsia (the gravest form of toxemia in pregnancy), ocular surgery, glaucoma, delirium tremens, epilepsy..."*

Researchers reported that they were undertaking further extensive research studies on the medical applications of urea.

Report #19   TITLE: *BACTERICIDAL EFFECT OF UREA,* 1961, by J.U. Schlegel, Jorge Cuellar and R.M. O'Dell, From Tulane University, School of Medicine, Department of Surgery, Division of Urology, New Orleans, Louisiana. This research was supported by Public Health Service Grants and Abbott Laboratories.

SUBJECT: UREA AND URINARY TRACT INFECTIONS.

Drawing on earlier historical research into urea's anti-bacterial properties, Schlegel and his associates conducted this study to determine what effect urea would have on bacteria commonly found in urinary tract infections such as bladder and kidney infections:

"It has been known since 1906 that urea has a bacteriostatic effect in altering the shape of pathogenic organisms (Peju and Rajat and Wilson).

Symmers and Kirk in 1915 used urea powder as a disinfectant in the treatment of wounds. It has also been used locally for preventing the spread of disease in surgery. Foshay (1935) used urea locally in otitis (ear infections) with good results.

McKay and Schroeder (1936) experimented with the use of urea on polio and rabies viruses and found that the viruses were weakened and finally destroyed by urea. Holder and Mackay (1943) used urea locally to stimulate new tissue in wounds and to remove dead tissue...

Weinstein and McDonald (1945) showed the bactericidal effect of urea on microorganisms...It was shown to be effective against typhoid, paratyphoid and dysentery bacilli...

Based on these findings, we proceeded to study the effect of urea in concentrations within physiological ranges on certain bacteria commonly found in urinary tract infections."

Even though they were unable to determine the mechanism whereby urea inhibited or killed the bacteria, Schlegel and his associates did conclude that:

"From the results obtained, it would appear that urea had a bacteriostatic or bactericidal effect on all organisms tested...As would be expected, the higher concentrations of urea and longer exposure were more effective."

This point is important because it demonstrates that as we increase the urea concentrations in our urine, we increase the germ-fighting properties of our urine, which is an important function of the body in resisting or defeating bacterial invasions as in bladder and kidney infections.

So how do we increase our bodies' urea levels? As the following study by Dr. Donald Kaye demonstrated, one way is by taking urea orally or by injection, as patients in his clinical trials did; another method is by ingesting our own urine, which, because it naturally contains urea, also increases urea concentrations in our systems.

One popular conventional medical treatment for urinary tract infections that does not increase urea levels, but actually dilutes urea, is the practice of force-drinking copious amounts of water or liquids to supposedly help cure urinary tract infections. This practice of force-drinking water to increase urine excretion is called water diuresis.

As Schlegel, and other researchers and clinical trials demonstrated, concentrated urine is actually a vital natural defense against urinary tract infections, including kidney infections, and diluting it by greatly increased forced-water intake is apparently an erroneous practice.

As Schlegel and his associates commented:

> *"Water diuresis results in urea concentration in urine so low that there would be no bactericidal effect due to urea.*
>
> *One consequently wonders about the rationale of instituting water diuresis by forced water intake as supportive therapy in acute pyelonephritis [kidney infection] or other urinary tract infections."*

In other words, Schlegel is saying that it isn't logical to drink large amounts of water to combat urinary tract infections, because the water dilutes the urine and its urea content which subsequently destroys or greatly decreases the urine's natural anti-bacterial action which the body uses as a natural defense against urinary tract infection.

Schlegel also observed that chronic kidney infection is associated with an inability to concentrate urine. This means that the kidney infection may be fueled by the fact that the urine or urea in the system isn't concentrated enough to exert its anti-bacterial action, and consequently can't help fight the infection:

> *"This finding helps to confirm that with a loss of ability to concentrate urine and the accompanying loss of ability to concentrate urea, as seen*

in advanced chronic pyelonephritis [kidney infection], the anti-bacterial concentration of urea cannot be achieved."

As Schlegel comments, when the body's urea concentration is diluted by such things as drinking large quantities of water or by kidney malfunction, the body loses its important natural capacity to use urea as an anti-bacterial defense.

Researchers have also discovered that acidic urine is more anti-bacterial than non-acidic urine. But again, drinking water large amounts of water makes urine less acidic and therefore less anti-bacterial.

In the book *Urinalysis in Clinical Laboratory Practice* written in 1975 by two researchers from Miles Laboratories, the researchers also observe that by drinking large amounts of water, the natural anti-bacterial-promoting acidity of urine is destroyed:

> *"If a large amount of water is ingested by a human, a corresponding diuresis or increase in urine excretion occurs. At this time, the pH of the urine tends to become relatively fixed at a value quite close to neutrality. **This phenomenon may be interpreted as an indication that the normal process of urine pH adjustment does not have an opportunity to function effectively...**"*

The researchers also stated that:

> *"The presence of a urinary tract infection may cause the urine to become quite definitely and persistently alkaline due to the action of urea splitting organisms."*

In other words, an infection itself makes the urine less acid and therefore less anti-bacterial than it should be, so logically, it doesn't make sense to further dilute the urine's bacteria-fighting properties by drinking large amounts of water as a treatment for the infection.

Cranberry juice has been suggested as a method for increasing the anti-bacterial acidity of urine, but as the next study by Dr. Donald Kaye demonstrated, the urea concentration and not the acidity of the urine appears to be the primary factor in urine's antibacterial activity, and force-drinking fluids does not contribute to urea concentration in the urine.

For women who have or have had urinary tract infections, more commonly referred to as bladder infections, you know what your doctor invariably tells you to do – drink lots of fluids and take medication, right?

But there are two major problems with this scenario. First, as we've discussed, drinking large amounts of fluid dilutes the antibacterial activity of your urine which makes it harder for your body to overcome the urinary tract infection.

Secondly, one of the medications which doctors invariably prescribe for the pain associated with bladder infections is Pyridium, (phenazopyridine hydrochloride). Unfortunately, Pyridium is a known carcinogen.

The *1985 Handbook of Toxic and Hazardous Chemicals and Carcinogens* states that Pyridium, (also known as Bisteril, Pyridicil and Uridinal), which has been used for 40 years as an analgesic drug to reduce the pain of urinary tract infections, is actually a known carcinogen:

> *"...in female mice it significantly increased the incidence of adenomas and carcinomas (cancer), and...In male and female rats it induced tumors of the colon and rectum."*

4.4 million prescriptions of this drug were dispensed in 1980, and it is still routinely prescribed for the pain of urinary tract infections today.

The next time you get a urinary tract infection, try urine therapy first – it's indisputably safer, cheaper, and much more effective than water, cranberry juice and Pyridium. And you can monitor your own progress at home with the same dipsticks the doctors use to determine if you have a urinary tract infection (see section on urine testing you can do at home in Chapter 6.)

The next research study was also done on the role of urine in preventing or healing urinary tract infections, and it also demonstrated that urine can inhibit or kill bacteria when the urea concentration is sufficiently elevated.

TITLE: *ANTIBACTERIAL ACTIVITY OF HUMAN URINE,* 1968, by Dr. Donald Kaye (Associate Professor of Medicine, Cornell University Medical College, New York).

Report #20

Many researchers in the past have looked for the answer as to why urine from one person is anti-bacterial, while a urine sample from another individual is not. Several studies over the course of the twentieth century confirmed that urine can definitely be anti-bacterial and, based on a number of these studies, researchers speculated that increased acid levels in urine made it antibacterial (which is the reason why cranberry juice, which acidifies the urine, is recommended for urinary tract infections).

But, Dr. Donald Kaye disagreed that acidity was the major factor in making urine anti-bacterial. He felt that, although acidity contributed to urine's anti-bacterial properties, no one had yet confirmed the real factor behind this natural activity of urine.

So in 1968 he undertook a research study in order to demonstrate that the bactericidal properties of urine were related not so much to acidity or other factors, but more to the urea concentration in the urine.

In the study, Kaye showed that it was primarily urea levels, rather than organic acids or other factors that were responsible for the antibacterial action of urine:

> *"The results of the present study provide evidence for the role of urea in human urine as an antibacterial agent.*
>
> *They also suggest that within the ranges of concentration commonly achieved in human urine, antibacterial activity is more a function of urea content than of organic acid concentration, or ammonium concentration."*

Kaye demonstrated that by increasing the concentration of urea in urine, you could directly increase the urine's ability to stop the growth of the disease-causing bacteria:

> *"...These experiments demonstrated that supplementation with urea markedly increased the inhibitory quality of the urine..."*

Kaye also mentions several other researchers who had demonstrated that concentrated urea was anti-bacterial:

> *"There are previous studies suggesting that urea may contribute to antibacterial activity of urine...Schlegel, Cuellar and O'Dell found that urea in nutrient broth...has antibacterial activity in concentrations of 1-4 g/100 ml...*
>
> *Neter and Clark showed that addition of urea to human urine markedly increased antibacterial activity.*
>
> *Finally, Schlegel, Raffi, Flinner, and O'Dell, Brazil, and Schlegel were able to decrease the incidence of urinary tract infection in dogs and rats by administering urea after introduction of bacteria into the urinary tract."*

When you re-ingest your urine, you are essentially ingesting additional urea. And as Kaye demonstrated in his study, by orally ingesting additional urea, we increase the concentration of urea in the system, and consequently increase the antibacterial action of our urine:

> *"Urine collected from volunteers after ingestion of urea demonstrated a marked increase in antibacterial activity, as compared with urine collected before ingestion of urea...*
>
> *In each subject the urea concentration was increased by at least 0.5 grams of urea nitrogen/100ml of urine after ingestion of urea."*

There is evidence that there is a link between acidity in urine and its antibacterial action, but, as Kaye comments:

> *"None of the studies made an intensive effort to elucidate the factors that may contribute to inhibitory activity of urine and to determine the relative importance of each factor."*

Kaye also demonstrates, as did Schlegel, that drinking large amounts of water to promote urine output (diuresis) markedly decreases the antibacterial activity of urine, which in turn decreases one of your body's natural infection-fighting mechanisms:

> *"Urine...collected before diuresis was bactericidal for E. Coli strain 14, whereas urine obtained during diuresis supported the growth of this strain...*
>
> *The results of the present study and those of Roberts and Beard and Asscher et al. suggest that antibacterial activity of human urine may be an important factor in preventing urinary tract infection and may also help to select (affect the reproduction of) bacterial strains when infection does occur."*

In view of all this supportive data on the antibacterial properties of urea, it becomes clearer as to why urine therapy has long been observed to be extremely effective in combatting many different types of infection.

Report #21   **TITLE:** *NEUTRALIZING ANTIBODY TO POLIOVIRUSES IN NOR-MAL HUMAN URINE,* 1962, by Martin Lerner, Jack Remington and Maxwell Finland, Journal of Clinical Investigation. (From the Throndike Memorial Laboratory, Harvard Medical Services, Boston City Hospital, and the Department of Medicine, Harvard Medical School, Boston Massachusetts, Journal of Clinical Investigation.

SUBJECT: NATURAL ANTIBODIES FOUND IN URINE

The research in this study was based in large part on several previous studies on the presence of important natural antibodies that have been found in urine.

Actually, there are so many research studies that have been done on the presence of antibodies in urine that it would be impossible to discuss them all, so we'll look at this study and one other, both of which give a good general overview of the subject.

We all know the importance of anti-bodies in fighting disease. When we are exposed to foreign organisms which our bodies sense as threatening, our immune system produces a wide variety of antibodies which attack, weaken and destroy the intruders.

Most of us think that these antibodies are found only in our blood. But numerous research studies have proven that a wide variety of antibodies are also present in our urine when we are fighting disease – and these important antibodies can be reused by the body in urine therapy.

As this study in 1962 revealed, urine antibodies are extremely effective disease-fighters and are capable of actively neutralizing or destroying even the aggressive polio virus:

> *Neutralizing activity for the poliovirus was demonstrated in protein concentrates prepared from the urine of a number of normal subjects. The biologic characteristics of the neutralizing activity in the urine resembled those of specific antibody found in blood.*
>
> **This neutralizing substance of the urine has the essential characteristics of antibody.** *Further studies on the biochemical and physical characterization of this and other urinary antibodies are in progress.*

This report also revealed that several other types of urine anti-bodies have been found in other research studies:

"Antibodies to cholera and typhoid have been found in the unconcentrated urine of normal volunteers immunized with the corresponding vaccine.

Antibodies to diphtheria, pneumonia, leptospira and salmonella bacteria have also been found in the urine of immunized or infected individuals."

The medical community may argue that the re-use of urine antibodies through urine therapy isn't significant because antibodies aren't always found in urine during disease and they are not sufficiently concentrated enough to control or combat disease even when they are found – but this isn't true.

The researchers in this study on polio urine antibodies clearly stated that even minute concentrations of detected or undetected antibodies can control and fight disease:

"It is known, however, that the presence of antibody, even in amounts which are not detectable by conventional methods, may prevent disease and detection of virus...".

In another research report published in 1967 by immunologists from Mount Sinai Hospital in New York on the presence of polioantibody in urine, the researchers confirmed that:

"It is clear that IGA polioantibody is present in...urine...It seems likely that antibodies of this type may play a part in the defense against invasion of micro-organisms." (Demonstration of IgA Polioantibody in Saliva, Duodenal Fluid and Urine, 1967)."

In other words, as these two studies demonstrate, natural urine antibodies do not necessarily need to be chemically concentrated in drug form in order to be active and effective, and, as we've seen, natural substances in their natural environment are safer and less toxic to use, which means that reusing urine antibodies through urine therapy is extremely significant.

Another important aspect of reusing urine antibodies during urine therapy that I've mentioned before is the fact that your urine antibodies are specific to your particular health conditions. When you reingest your urine, you get the benefit of your body's "custom-made" antibodies to combat diseases you may not even know you have.

The recent outbreaks of food poisoning from contaminated beef and chicken presents an important indication for the use of urine and urea therapy. Urine, as you've read, contains natural antibodies to food contaminants such as salmonella in infected individuals, and many people have reported excellent success in treating food poisoning with urine therapy. Also, concentrated urea's excellent bactericidal properties can also contribute to treating bacterial infections such as food poisoning.

In serious, hospitalized cases, the administration of the patient's urine combined with injected or intravenous urea would provide a combination of natural antibodies, critical immune defense factors and concentrated urea levels that could prove to be of enormous efficacy in treating food poisoning and bacterial and viral infections of all kinds.

As a nation, we spend an enormous amount of time and money trying to diagnose what disorders we have and usually end up with an antibiotic or drug that may or may not be the right one for our 'non-specific' illness. Urine therapy provides an alternative to this practice, because we don't have to diagnose every condition we have in order for it to be effective.

Urine therapy is completely safe and applicable to a huge variety of conditions, in addition to being an excellent preventative health treatment. There are many instances when your immune system is dealing with a health threat long before overt symptoms appear. With urine therapy, however, urine antibodies, hormones, enzymes and extremely complex nutritional elements can help combat illnesses before symptoms appear and even before they're detectable by conventional diagnostic studies.

Report #22 **TITLE:** *USE OF EXOGENOUS AND ENDOGENOUS UREA FOR PROTEIN SYNTHESIS IN NORMAL AND UREMIC SUBJECTS,* 1963, by Dr. Carmelo Giordano, from the Renal Laboratory, Naples University School of Medicine.

This study has to do with one of the most difficult problems in renal, or kidney disorders, which is the patient's impaired ability to synthesize, or in other words, break down and use protein. Protein is normally broken down into nitrogen and other constituents by both the liver and the kidneys, but when the kidneys malfunction because of infection, damage, etc. and can't break down protein efficiently, protein depletion occurs, nitrogen levels are altered in the body and the person's health is severely threatened.

However, some researchers, such as Giordano, have discovered that urea, (which is produced during protein synthesis and therefore contains nitrogen), can actually play a role in helping kidney patients to use protein more efficiently and to achieve proper nitrogen balance in the body.

The study demonstrated that:

> *"If urea was added to the diet, enough synthesis of nonessential amino acids occurred to achieve equilibrium or even positive nitrogen balance."*

As Giordano points out:

> *"With the use of a synthetic diet containing essential amino acids in low quantity, it is shown that urea, either if given exogenously or if taken endogenously from waste nitrogen retained in uremia, is utilized for the synthesis of non-essential amino acids."*

Utilization of urea has shown progressive clinical improvement in uremic patients and is under study as a treatment of renal [kidney] failure.

Another report on the role of urea in kidney disease was delivered at an international symposium in Florida in 1968, entitled Urea and the Kidney, In the report, Mackenzie Walser, of the Johns Hopkins University School of Medicine, stated that:

> *"In uremics [kidney patients] on diets containing small amounts of protein, urea apparently provides the principal source of nitrogen for protein synthesis. Further exploration of these findings may yield valuable information in the treatment of renal failure."*

Walser also points out that:

> ***Urea can no longer be regarded as an end-product of nitrogen metabolism but may be used for protein synthesis.***

In other words, studies have shown that urea is not just a "waste" or by-product of the body's use of protein, but is actually an important part of our bodies' process of metabolizing protein and maintaining proper nitrogen levels which are critical to health and functioning.

Report #23   TITLE: *CHARACTERIZATION OF ANTIBODIES IN HUMAN URINE*, 1965, by Lars A. Hanson and Eng M. Tan, (From the Rockefeller Institute, N.Y., N.Y.). published in the *Journal of Clinical Investigation.*

This study is another research project done on antibodies in human urine and was presented by Dr. Lars A. Hanson of the Pediatric Clinic of the Karolinska Institute in Sweden at the meeting of the Microbiology Section of the Swedish Medical Society in Stockholm.

The report stated that:

> *Human urine contains proteins that have been shown to be identical with serum (blood) immunoglobulin or (antibodies).*

The report also revealed that:

> *Antibody activity in urine has been demonstrated against several microorganisms including* **cholera, salmonella, diphtheria, tetanus and polio.**

Many of the doctors who used urine therapy on patients early in the twentieth century such as Duncan, and Plesch noted that the ingestion or injection of an individual's own urine had an often amazing curative effect on a surprisingly wide variety of bacterial and viral-related illnesses such as hepatitis, whooping cough, mumps, chicken pox and influenza.

It's interesting to see that modern medical researchers have confirmed the presence of a variety of disease antibodies in urine that apparently play a role in the successful clinical applications of urine therapy.

There are many other references to urine antibodies in medical literature, a few more of which I will list here.

The gammaglobulins which are mentioned in the report titles are extremely important immune defense antibody factors:

> *Blood group antibodies in human urine.*
> **Prager and Bearden**
> **Transfusion, 1965**

> *Further studies of the gamma related proteins of normal urine.*
> **Journal of Clinical Investigation, 1962**

Characterization of antibodies in normal human urine by gel-filtration and antigenic analysis.
M.W. Turner
Protides of the Biological Fluids, 1964

Proteins, glycoproteins and mucopolysaccharides in normal human urine.
I. Berggard
Arkiv. Kemi, 1961

An unusual micro-gamma-globulin in the serum and urine of a patient.
Franklin, Meltzer, Guggenhein and Lowenstein
Fed. Proc., 1963

Physiochemical and immunologic studies of gamma globulins of normal human urine.
E.C. Franklin
Journal of Clinical investigation, 1959

Significance of urinary gamma globulin in lupus nephritis.
Stevens and Knowles
New England Journal of Medicine, 1962

It's extraordinary to realize that we have such easy access to these extremely important natural antibodies and other critical immune elements of the blood through the simple use of urine therapy – especially in view of the AIDS scare which makes the use of any public source of blood-related medical treatments frightening to many people today.

TITLE: *NATURE AND COMPOSITION OF URINE FROM HEALTHY SUBJECTS*, 1975, by A.H. Free., H.M. Free, from Urinalysis in Clinical Laboratory Practice, Miles Laboratories.   *Report #1*

SUBJECT: INGREDIENTS OF NORMAL HUMAN URINE

In general, most of us have no idea that urine is an extraordinary body fluid derived from the blood that is filled with hundreds of health supporting ingredients – but, for that matter, this is a fact that scientists themselves have only begun to fully understand within the last few decades.

As Free and Free explain:

> *"Literally thousands of compounds have been identified in normal urine and the vast majority of these have been derived from the blood...*
>
> *The understanding of the composition of the urine has gradually evolved as the sciences of chemistry and physiology have developed...*
>
> *It is now recognized that the urine contains thousands of compounds, and as new, more sensitive analytical tools evolve; it is quite certain that new constituents of urine will be recognized."*

This report goes on to give a detailed listing of approximately 200 constituents of urine, but as the researchers comment: *this table is not considered to be complete, but identifies [only] compounds of interest."*

Listing all 200 of the ingredients here would be a bit much, so I'll give a sample of some of the ingredients in urine that are most recognizable because many of them are the same ingredients that you see on your vitamin supplement labels, or that you've read or heard about from various sources.

Again, we never think of urine as a nutrient, but as this analysis of urine shows, there are numerous elements of nutritional value in urine, along with hormones, steroids, and other critical elements that regulate and control key processes of the body:

Alanine, total	.38 mg/day	Lysine, total	.56 mg/day
Arginine, total	.32 mg/day	Magnesium	100 mg/day
Ascorbic acid	.30 mg/day	Manganese	0.5 mg/day
Allantoin	.12 mg/day	Methionine, total	10 mg/day
Amino acids, total	.2.1 g/day	Nitrogen, total	15 g/day
Bicarbonate	140 mg/day	Ornithine	10 mg/day
Biotin	.35 mg/day	Pantothenic acid	3 mg/day
Calcium	.23 mg/day	Phenylalanine	.21 mg/day
Creatinine	1.4 mg/day	Phosphorus, organic	.9 mg/day
Cystine	120 mg/day	Potassium	2.5 mg/day
Dopamine	0.40 mg/day	Proteins, total	.35 mg/day
Epinephrine	0.01 mg/day	Riboflavin	0.9 mg/day
Folic acid	.4 mg/day	Tryptophan, total	.28 mg/day
Glucose	100 mg/day	Tyrosine, total	.50 mg/day
Glutamic Acid	308 mg/day	Urea	24.5 mg/day
Glycine	455 mg/day	Vitamin B6	100 mg/day
Inositol	.14 mg/day	Vitamin B12	0.03 mg/day
Iodine	0.25 mg/day	Zinc	1.4 mg/day
Iron	0.5 mg/day		

Hormonal Substances

Aldosterone, male . . . . .3.5 mg/day	Estriol, female
Aldosterone, female . . .4.2 mg/day	luteal phase . . . . .28 mg/day
	Estrone, female
Androgens, female	luteal phase . . . . .14 mg/day
(20-40 yrs.) . . . . .14 mg/day	
Androgens, male	17-Ketogenic adrenocoriticoids
(20-40 yrs.) . . . . .18.2 mg/day	female . . . . .12.6 mg/day
	17-Ketogenic adrenocoriticoids
Androsterone, female . .4.2 mg/day	male . . . . .14.7 mg/day
Androsterone, male . . . .3.5 mg/day	
	Ketol steroids . . . . . . .18.2 mg/day
Estradiol, female	
luteal phase . . . . .7 mg/day	

An interesting point about many of these urine ingredients is that many of them are naturally synthesized forms of key nutritional elements. For instance, the synthesized, or "digested" forms of vitamin B6 (pyridoxine) are found in urine – Pyridoxal (70 mg/day) and Pyridoxamine (100 mg/day). When you ingest B6 (pyridoxine) in your food or as a vitamin supplement, the body breaks it down into simpler substances that it can use, namely, pyridoxal and pyridoxamine.

These two substances have tremendous nutritive value. They're essential for the synthesis and breakdown of amino acids, the conversion of tryptophan to niacin, the breakdown of glycogen to glucose, the production of antibodies, the formation of heme in hemoglobin, the formation of hormones important in brain function, the proper absorption of B12, and the maintenance of the balance of sodium and potassium which regulates body fluids.

In using natural urine therapy, you are not only ingesting B6 itself, but you are also ingesting the already synthesized forms of B6, which can be extremely important to people who have an impaired ability to utilize B vitamins or other essential nutrients in their systems due to such factors as poor digestion and assimilation, aging, the use of drugs, oral contraceptives, antibiotics, etc.

There are many "pre-digested" nutritional products on the market today for people whose bodies have a difficult time breaking down more complex nutritional substances into elements that the body can use efficiently. But urine in itself is an incredibly complex and complete mixture of your own already pre-synthesized nutrients that no chemist anywhere could ever duplicate.

As a matter of fact, Bjornesjo, the researcher who did the studies on the anti-tuberculin activity of urine, did conduct experiments using an artificial urine concocted in the laboratory. **He found, however, that whereas natural urine did kill or stop the growth of the TB bacteria, the artificial urine did not, because the natural anti-TB urine element could not be synthetically duplicated.**

Several of the following research reports deal specifically with urine therapy treatments of cancer, AIDS, mental disorders, skin conditions and urea's dermatological and cosmetic uses, and these particular reports have been grouped in sections under their appropriate category titles to make it easier for you to review them.

URINE THERAPY AND CANCER

Report #25   **TITLE:** *H-11 FOR CANCER,* by Dr. J.H. Thompson, 1943, published in the *British Medical Journal,* (7/31/43).

In the late 1930's and early 40's, many medical researchers such as Dr. Thompson, were experimenting with an anti-cancer urine extract referred to as H-11.

Many of the hundreds of researchers who had conducted the studies on H-11 in cancer treatments over approximately a 12-year period experienced excellent results which unfortunately were ignored by the medical community. The researchers reportedly demanded that a medical research council be set up to review their complaints, stating that their research findings on successful H-11 cancer treatments were being unjustly ignored by the medical establishment. A council was set up in 1948, However, despite thousands of laboratory studies and hundreds of cases of clinical proof demonstrating the efficacy of H-11 in treating cancer, it was set aside by the council as an accepted medical treatment for cancer.

The clinical and laboratory findings on the use of this extract on cancer patients was reported in the *British Medical Journal* by Dr. J.H. Thompson, and revealed that over 300 independent doctors and researchers had found that H-11 was clinically effective in inhibiting the growth of malignant cells in humans.

TITLE: *THERAPEUTIC RESULTS OF THE USE OF AN AUTO-URINE EXTRACT ON MALIGNANT TUMORS,* 1961, by Dr. Novak, published in the German journal, *Zeitschrift Innere Medizine,* (Journal of Internal Medicine).

Report #26

This is an extremely interesting report from a German doctor who utilized injections of a natural urine extract prepared from each patients' own urine to treat several different types of cancer including stomach, colon, rectal, breast, lung, uterine, lymph node and gall bladder malignancies.

The results were remarkable in the majority of the 21 cases treated, and the report includes x-ray photos that corroborate the results. As an example:

CASE #2:   A 60 year-old woman with metastatic malignant tumors in the epigastrium and liver was treated with the urine extract. After 4 injections, both subjective and objective improvement was noted, as corroborated by radiological x-rays showing marked tumor reduction. After six weeks, there were no obstructions noted in the upper abdomen and the liver was normal. Two years have passed since the treatments and there has been no further incidence of the cancer.

CASE #3:   52-year-old woman with jaundice (serum bilirubin 11 mg.%). Melon-sized tumor in the right epi- and mesogastrium; exploratory laparotomy revealed advanced cancer of the gallbladder with metastases to the liver, cecum and transverse colon. After 5 injections of the urine extract, there was shrinkage of the tumor, reduction in size of the liver, bilirubin dropped to 1.6 mg%. Within 10 months of follow-up examinations, the patient exhibited no symptoms; on rare occasions, stomach upset occurred after dietary irregularities.

Report #27   **TITLE:** *PREPARATION OF RETINE FROM HUMAN URINE,* by Albert Szent-Gyorgi, et.al., 1963, published in Science Magazine. Study supported by grants from the National Institute of Health and the National Science Foundation and conducted at the Institute for Muscle Research, in Massachusetts.

SUBJECT: EFFECTS OF A URINE EXTRACT ON MALIGNANT CANCER TUMORS

This study was done on an anti-cancer element that has been extracted from urine called "retine":

"Certain fractions of the urine of children have been shown to stop the growth of transplanted malignant cancer tumors in mice. The substance responsible for this action was called "retine". We have since found a similar activity in the urine of adults of about 20-25 years."

After studying the effect of retine on several different types of cancerous tumors, the researchers observed that:

"Smaller doses of retine inhibit growth of the tumors, while bigger ones actually make the tumors regress."

In the study, a group of mice were injected under the skin with 30 million live cancer cells, and developed subsequent tumors. The mice were then treated with retine for a week and the researchers noted that:

"The tumors of the mice treated with 6 units of retine for a week, upon examination, were found to contain very little live cancer tissue and consisted chiefly of dead cancer cells."

Unfortunately, retine has not been publicized as an anti-cancer agent, but this study, as do others, demonstrates that there are important anti-cancer factors in urine that have been shown to be amazingly effective in destroying and stopping the growth of malignant cancerous tumors and cells.

TITLE: *TREATMENT OF GASTRIC CANCER WITH HUD, AN ANTI-GENIC SUBSTANCE OBTAINED FROM PATIENT'S URINE,* 1968, by Dr. Momoe Soeda, Tokyo, Japan.

This research report presents the remarkable results of a cancer treatment study utilizing a urine derivative called HUD (Human's Urine Derivative). HUD was found in significant amounts in the urine of cancer patients and was shown to have distinct anti-cancer properties:

> *"A variety of people were tested and it was found that the urine of cancer patients almost invariably contains a considerable amount of a natural immune defense substance named HUD (Human's Urine Derivative).*
>
> *HUD was clinically applied to an intractable case of metastatic (spreading) ovarian cancer in June, 1965 and we were very impressed with its excellent effect on regression of metastatic tumors."*

After the HUD treatment was applied the researchers noted that:

> ***"Almost all metastases completely disappeared during a course of 3 months after the start of HUD therapy, and the patient was discharged under a quite favorable condition. More than 30 months have passed since she was discharged and now she is completely well and enjoying the rest of her life."***

HUD therapy was also applied to several patients with gastric cancer after surgery in order to prevent the common post-surgical reoccurrence of the cancer:

> *"8 patients were treated with HUD immediately after operation. In 5 cases in this group, the cancer had invaded the stomach wall and involved the lymph nodes. The postoperative prognosis for this group of patients was very poor, and their 3-year survival rate was considered to less than 40 percent.*
>
> *However, following HUD treatments, 3 years passed and 7 out of the 8 patients treated are completely well and participating in almost full activities without any signs of recurrence.*
>
> *In view of these facts it is apparent that HUD is effective in suppressing the post-operative recurrence of gastric cancer and that such effect may presumably be due to its ability to reinforce the immune system of the cancer patient."*

These researchers also commented on the danger and ineffectiveness of radiation and chemotherapy in the treatment of cancer:

> *"Radiation therapy and anti-cancer chemotherapy have been extensively tested for many years to control postoperative spreading and growth of tumor cells, however, it may be fairly said that both measures have almost completely failed this purpose up to the present time."*

The researchers comment on the extreme importance of maintaining the integrity of the immune system in treating cancer and they discuss how radiation and chemo destroy the immunological defenses of the body, especially plasma cells which are involved in antibody production and natural resistance to cancer. The report recommends that:

> *"Emphasis should be placed on discovering anti-cancer agents, such as HUD which exert an inhibitory effect on malignant cells without damaging the body's natural immune defenses."*

A reinforcement of this medical opinion on the ineffectiveness of chemotherapy is another study done in 1985 which was published in Scientific American and stated that:

> *"Only 2 to 5 percent of cancer deaths are prevented by chemotherapeutic drugs, and their side effects are devastating."*
> **— Informed Consumers Pharmacy**

As research suggests, preserving and reinforcing the immune system during cancer treatment is critical. The researchers in this study on HUD noted that patients with inoperable, advanced cases of gastric cancer whose immune systems were severely damaged often did not improve after HUD therapy.

But here again is an example of how natural urine therapy could been of more assistance than an isolated urine extract. The HUD extract is only one infinitesimal fraction out of hundreds of immune defense factors and other proven anti-cancer agents which whole urine contains. So these advanced cancer patients treated with HUD received only one single beneficial urine element when they could have been receiving the full range of benefits that whole urine has to offer. Perhaps, ideally, clinical treatments of cancer could incorporate natural urine therapy, augmented by the administration of concentrated urine extracts to enhance healing.

Many cancer patients who have successfully used natural urine therapy to treat their cancer have reported it to be a safe and effective cancer treatment which rids the body of cancerous manifestations while at the same time greatly enhancing the immune system. But in consideration of all of the nutrients, enzymes, antibodies and other immune defense factors such as retine or HUD that urine contains, it's not surprising that it has been found by many to be such an effective cancer treatment.

TITLE: *ANTINEOPLASTON A IN CANCER THERAPY,* 1977, by Stanislaw R. Burzynski et. al, published in Physiological Chemistry and Physics, a publication that reports fundamental new research in biochemistry and biophysics.

Report #29

This report is one of many published by Dr. Burzynski on anti-cancer agents which he discovered in human urine called "antineoplastons". In this and many succeeding laboratory and clinical studies on antineoplastons, Burzynski demonstrated remarkable success in treating various types of cancer with these urine extracts:

> *"In recent years we were able to describe a number of peptide fractions [proteins], isolated from normal human urine, that produce remarkable inhibition of...various neoplastic cells [cancer tumors] without showing significant inhibition in normal cells...In our experiments we chose normal human urine as the most economical source for the isolation of antineoplastons."*

Burzynski's work using antineoplastons in cancer treatment, which has been suppressed by the conventional medical establishment, brings up the huge issue of alternative cancer therapies. This is an enormous subject and not one which can be examined in great detail here without straying miles down the road from the subject of urine therapy.

But the fact is, that if you have cancer, you absolutely need to read the arguments against conventional treatments with radiation and chemotherapy – and there are many convincing ones, such as the last report on HUD in which medical researchers themselves discourage the use of toxic and generally ineffective accepted cancer treatments such as chemotherapy and radiation.

In 1979, Gary Null, a famous New York City talk show host and consumer advocate, published a series of excellent articles on the suppression of cancer cures in the U.S.

One of the cancer treatments that has been suppressed involves the use of these antineoplastons that naturally occur in urine, discovered by Dr.

Burzynski. Gary Null, interviewed Burzynski in October 1979 and revealed hidden facts on Antineoplaston A:

"We can see how the cancer blackout works by looking at the case of a young Polish doctor named Stanislaw Burzynski. In the past few years, this doctor has published ten papers on the positive results of a substance called antineoplaston a on certain types of tumors. One of the youngest men in his native country to hold an M.D. and a Ph.D degree, Dr. Burzynski found life under communism difficult and decided to come to the United States to seek more freedom for his scientific research...

Documented cases of spontaneous remission and prolonged cancer arrest in humans led Dr. Burzynski to consider how the body might fight cancer on its own. The body must have some way, he thought, to correct errors that occur in cellular differentiation and to redirect potential cancer cells into normal paths. The theory is, of course, that cancer cells have lost the 'information' needed to develop into differentiated body-organ cells.

Burzynski's antineoplaston a allegedly supplies that 'information' in the form of a protein peptide, (a chain of amino acids) – one of the best biological information carriers – that would reprogram cancer cells into normal growth.

Although antineoplastons are found in all normal body tissues and fluids, THEY ARE MOST EASILY EXTRACTED FROM URINE (my caps). They appear to "normalize" cancer cells without inhibiting the growth of normal cells.

Actually, urine therapy has been used as folk remedy for cancer and other ailments for over 2,000 years. Even within the past 30 years, at least 45,000 injections of urine or urine extract were given in the United States and throughout Europe without any toxic side effects."

In reality, unknown to Gary Null and most of us, there have been several hundred thousand oral administrations and injections of urine and urea given by doctors and researchers over the last 30 years. Null continues:

"In our search for antineoplastons, says Burzynski, 'we were able to find peptides in normal human urine...that were active against every type of human neoplasm (tumor) we tested, including myeloblastic leukemia, osteosarcoma, fibrosarcoma, chondrosarcoma, cancer of the uterine cervix, colon cancer, breast cancer, and lymphoma.'

Dr. Burzynski presented his startling results to the annual meeting of the Federation of the American Societies for Experimental Biology...

"However, soon after this Dr. Burzynski's funding was decreased, then it was discontinued. His work was channeled into other areas of research, and his superiors discouraged his pursuit of cancer therapy."

The article continues with details of the extraordinary results of Burzynski's treatment in one particular case:

"Working for the past two years in the relative freedom of his own lab, Dr. Burzynski has amassed some impressive results. For example, there was the case of a 63-year old white male with lung cancer that had spread to the brain. Before coming to Dr. Burzynski, the patient had received chemotherapy and cobalt treatment, whereby a part of the brain tumor had been reduced. However, a new tumor had sprung up in another part of his brain, and doctors decided that nothing more could be done. Undaunted, the patient's family searched out Dr. Burzynski, who examined the patient and cautiously agreed to help.

After just two weeks of the antine-oplaston treatment, in which the patient was given the substance intravenously, the tumor on the left lung decreased substantially. After six weeks it disappeared entirely. After a month both brain metastases decreased in size and, in six weeks, also disappeared. Amazingly, the only side effects of this highly effective treatment were chills and fever. These were attributed to the release of toxic products into the bloodstream after the breakdown of cancer cells. Contrast this with the deleterious effects of conventional therapy, which in this patient's case had increased the metastasis..."

Dr. Burzynski still uses his treatment successfully in his lab in Houston today, although he is continually assaulted by the medical society in Houston and has been refused research grants from the American Cancer Society and the National Cancer Institute – even though his findings on the anticancer properties of antineoplaston A have been confirmed in tests by prestigious research centers all over the U.S. on leukemia and other types of cancer, including breast cancer.

Urine extracts such as H-11, retine, HUD and antineoplastons, as the research has demonstrated, gave excellent results in treating cancer patients, but, again, these anti-cancer elements are already available in natural urine and can be simply, safely and easily accessed, whereas accessing urine extract treatments can be difficult and extremely expensive – and I know this from my own experience.

After several unsuccessful surgeries for endometriosis, I was told that I would need more surgery. After my doctor told me that he was scheduling another operation for me, I canceled the surgery and flew to Mexico to get an alternative treatment for cancer patients that I was told also had possibilities for treating my case.

The cancer clinics in Mexico reminded me of something out of Sartre – shaven-headed terminal cancer patients lined up by the dozens with IV tubes dangling from their arms, some of them with huge, ulcerated, open cancerous lesions oozing blood. The man in the bed next to mine had a cancerous brain tumor the size of a large grapefruit bulging from his head. One of his eyes, nearly eaten away by the cancer, was now just a mass of bloody, unrecognizable tissue.

But as I soon discovered, the people in the clinic were the "lucky" ones. As I sat listlessly in my chair with my IV tube pumping a $10,000.00 course of "immune builders" into my body, I watched as a steady procession of cancer patients came through the clinic, asking for information on other less expensive cancer treatments because they couldn't afford the fees for the alternative clinics.

The stories, most of which I could overhear, were all the same – these cancer victims had gone through months or years of radiation and chemo, the cancer was back, and now they were dying; they'd turned to natural medicine as a last resort, but couldn't afford the $10,000 to $50,000 that the alternative clinics charged.

These were hopeless, desperate people, many of them only in their twenties and thirties – but what could they do? Conventional medicine hadn't worked, they had no knowledge about natural therapies, no idea about how to help themselves – it was a scenario of gruesome and devastating personal ordeals that the American Cancer Society and the AMA never reveal.

And these people are not in the minority. It has been reported that:

> *"Nearly two-thirds of all cancer patients will eventually die of their diagnosed cancer, either before or after the arbitrary five-year limit."*
> **Betrayal of Health**

It's always bothered me that I didn't know about urine therapy at that time, because I saw so many people who could have benefitted so much from it. A young girl came into the clinic alone one day, and I happened to talk to her.

She was twenty-four and had been diagnosed with ovarian cancer which had not responded to aggressive surgery, radiation and chemo, and her doctors said there was nothing more they could do for her. Her parents couldn't help her financially, she wasn't married, couldn't work, and had no money of her own, so she was unable to pay for alternative treatments like the one I was receiving.

She told me that in desperation she had gotten into her car and driven from her home in the Midwest to Mexico in hopes of finding some help. She asked me if I knew of any place that she could buy laetrile – she thought that perhaps she could treat herself with it, but I was unable to help her.

The bleak look of hopeless despair on her face was horrifying, and I would have loved to have been able to hand her a book on urine therapy – it was something she could have used herself, for free, in her own home, that undoubtedly would have given her control over her health and, at the very least, an excellent fighting chance. After all, she had everything to gain and nothing to lose by using this safe, proven natural therapy.

The urine therapist of the 1930's and 40's, John Armstrong, recounts many stories of curing cancer with urine fasts, massages and compresses:

> *"And now I will mention the case of a lady who came to me in 1927. It is instructive as showing once again that operations merely deal with effects and do not remove the cause of the disease from the body. The lady in question was 45, and had a growth of some size in her left breast, the right one having been removed two years previously for a similar growth.*
>
> *She fasted and was treated according to my method for nineteen days, and then reported that the growth had entirely vanished...On the 28th day, there was no trace of the lump...*
>
> *Lady of 62; diagnosed cancer of the bowel. Colostomy advised by the profession but refused...after urine therapy, complete cure.*
>
> *Lady of 42, diagnosed cancer of the breast. Excision advised...but only faint hope of cure...Patient refused operation. Complete cure by the fasting-urine method. Is still alive and well after 21 years."*

Naturally Armstrong's experiences, having no scientific support, were completely ignored by the medical establishment. But it's interesting to discover that medical research later revealed significant anti-cancer elements in urine that are extremely effective in treating and healing a wide variety of cancers. This modern scientific evidence provides corroboration to Armstrong's experiences, illustrating that his cures were much more than figments of his imagination.

Cancer is a frightening disease, but with the assiduous and wise use of natural healing methods such as urine therapy, proper nutrition, herbs, rest, homeopathic remedies, etc., many have controlled and cured their cancer without resorting to methods which damage the immune system such as chemotherapy or radiation.

Before you resort to any conventional cancer treatment, go to your local library and research your case by reading material related to different treatment options. It's crucial to find out the real success statistics on conventional treatments – don't just blindly accept your oncologist's recommendations.

I have a close relative who learned this lesson the hard way. After surgery for colon cancer, she called me and said that her oncologist wanted her to take a follow-up course of chemotherapy, "just in case", even though the surgery had taken out all existing non-metastasized tumors. I told her what I had read about the extreme side effects, dangers and inadequacy of chemo, but under pressure from her oncologist, she took the "treatment".

Unfortunately, she had a severe allergic reaction to the chemicals, nearly died and spent several totally unnecessary and horribly painful weeks in the hospital recovering from the extremely harmful effects of the chemotherapy, some of which were irreversible.

The use of chemotherapy and radiation is so damaging and traumatic to the body and it's success rate is so low that it's difficult to understand why anyone would resort to it once they are made aware of the truth of its danger and inadequacy without first trying aggressive urine therapy and other forms of natural healing. Many doctors themselves are acutely aware of the futility and danger of the conventional cancer treatments:

> "In 1955, the late Dr. Hardin Jones, professor of medical physics at the University of California, after studying cancer statistics for the previous thirty-three years, concluded that **untreated cancer victims lived up to four times longer than treated individuals.**
>
> Dr. Jones pointed out that the cure rates most often cited by doctors were (and continue to be) based only on the conventional treatment of the most favorable cases. **If the less 'curable' cases were figured in,**

conventional therapies would emerge as having little, no, or even aggravating impact on cancer patients overall."
Betrayal of Health

A recent article in *Forbes Magazine* in June of 1993 entitled *"An Educated Consumer is the best patient"*, describes a woman, Janice Guthrie, who was diagnosed with a rare type of ovarian cancer (granulosa cell tumor). She had emergency surgery, and, to her consternation, her oncologist recommended radiation therapy as a follow-up:

> *"To regain some control of her life, Guthrie went straight to the University of Arkansas medical school library in Little Rock. 'I wanted to see what was involved in my treatment,' she says, and to try to counteract any of the negative side effects.' But in the course of her reading, Guthrie discovered that radiation therapy didn't keep granulosa patients alive any longer than those who opted for regular checkups after surgery. Guthrie's oncologist didn't think much of her research. 'You can know too much,' he warned. Recalls Guthrie, 'It really made me mad'.*

In the end, Guthrie ignored her oncologist and through her research, found a doctor at the M.D. Anderson Cancer Center in Houston who successfully helped her condition without radiation.

So become an educated consumer about your cancer, and above all, vigorously support your body's own natural defenses with excellent nutrition, rest, relaxation and assiduous, educated use of natural healing methods like herbs, homeopathy, and of course urine therapy.

The body has amazing curative powers of its own, and if we would simply support our natural healing powers rather than beating them down with toxic chemical interventions and poor health habits, our ability to overcome cancer would be greatly increased and the unnecessary suffering associated with accepted cancer treatments would be eradicated.

Report #30   **TITLE:** *DHEA: "MIRACLE" DRUG?* 1982, by Saul Kent, published in *Geriatrics*, September, 1982.

SUBJECT: AIDS, OBESITY, CANCER, AGING

This report deals with a substance which is found in large quantities in the urine called dehydroepiandrosterone or DHEA to us. DHEA is a hormone that is already present in the body, and is actually related to testosterone, a male hormone.

Within the last decade, scientists have been analyzing and experimenting with this hormone because it apparently has significant anti-cancer, anti-obesity and anti-aging properties and has even been used in AIDS treatment.

As Dr. Kent comments, DHEA has been found by researchers to have several different biologic actions in animal studies:

> *"DHEA was added to a culture medium containing two potent chemical carcinogens. It was discovered that DHEA was remarkably successful in protecting cultured rodent cells against the cancer-causing agents that were added to the cells."*

While studying the anti-cancer effects of DHEA, another researcher, Dr. Schwartz also reported that the experimental animals **gained much less weight** as they grew older than normal animals:

> *"Apparently, DHEA was keeping body weight down without suppressing appetite or restricting food intake...In one study [it was] found that DHEA could even prevent weight increase in mice genetically bred to become obese in adulthood."*

Further research also revealed that mice treated with DHEA had a much younger appearance, showing much less coarsening and graying of the hair than animals not receiving DHEA:

> *"This suggests that DHEA may have an anti-aging effect as well as anti-cancer and anti-obesity effects."*

Users of urine therapy have reported for years that they weighed less and looked remarkably younger after consistent use of urine therapy, so it's interesting to read these studies on DHEA in urine which most likely also plays a role in urine therapy's excellent success in treating cancer, obesity and aging.

Another important thing that was brought out in this report is that studies have shown that women with breast cancer have lower-than-normal levels of DHEA, sometimes for years before they even develop the cancer. So it certainly makes sense to supplement DHEA in the body, which you can do easily, safely and at no cost with urine therapy.

Uric acid, which was mentioned previously, has also been discovered to destroy free radicals which are thought to contribute to the development of cancer.

SUMMARY ON CANCER AND URINE THERAPY

Not only does urine contain innumerable easily assimilable nutrients, hormones, enzymes, anti-bacterial agents and antibodies that help support the immune system during cancer, but urine also contains proven anti-cancer agents such as:

- Human Urine's Derivative (HUD)
- H-11 Extract
- Retine
- Antineoplastons
- DHEA Hormone
- Uric Acid

Urine therapy is obviously an excellent natural cancer treatment. Its nutritional benefits alone are phenomenal, not to mention the immense value of its innumerable other health-promoting, therapeutic agents.

DETECTING CANCER THROUGH URINE TESTS

Another important thing to consider in terms of cancer diagnosis is the fact that research has shown that certain components of urine sediment can be of great importance in identifying bladder, kidney and prostrate malignancies. In 1975, it was reported that urine studies are done on all urology patients at the Mayo Clinic to help detect cancer:

"Cancer cells from early-stage urinary system tumors appear in the urine, which allows for detection of such new tumors before they are readily perceived by other diagnostic methods.

Cells of urine sediment have been used in the same way that vaginal smears have been used to gain information on ovarian functioning. As a matter of fact, it was reported in 1971 that urine testing was actually shown to detect more cases of abnormal cell activity than the usual cervical Pap smear.

Urine testing for urinary tract malignancies is a safe, easy procedure which can replace or supplement other forms of cancer detection."
Urinalysis in Clinical Laboratory Practice

This type of diagnosis is so important today because, as many doctors and patients are finding, cancer patients can actually be harmed by the diagnostic tests themselves.

URINE THERAPY AND AIDS

Report #31   ***RESEARCH INDICATIONS FOR AIDS***

As we've seen, DHEA, which is present in large amounts in urine has many diverse health applications and *has also been reported as an AIDS treatment.*

The January, 1988 publication of *Aids Treatment News*, had an excellent article on the use of DHEA in AIDS. The article stated that:

Researchers suspect that AIDS patients have abnormally low levels of DHEA. Additionally, it is now believed that DHEA itself may have a direct anti-viral effect.

With urine therapy, AIDS patients have easy, unlimited access to DHEA, which reportedly has been forced from the consumer market by the FDA for no apparent reason.

Raising DHEA levels in the body through internal urine therapy certainly is a safe, simple procedure that both cancer and AIDS patients can undoubtedly benefit from. But DHEA is only one of, as we have seen, many hundreds of vitally important immune boosting and health supporting elements in urine.

Because of urine (and urea's) remarkable anti-viral properties, and its extraordinary capacity to heal and strengthen the immune system, it's obviously an immensely significant natural treatment for AIDS.

Actually, urine therapy in treating AIDS has already been in the news, although it's still not widely known or accepted because, up until now, the scientific evidence and proof supporting the efficacy of urine therapy has never been compiled and publicly presented.

An article done on AIDS treatments in 1988 in the magazine, *SPIN*, discusses the use of urine therapy in AIDS:

> *"One of the latest and most interesting treatments for which the alternative community is holding a lot of hope is probably the oldest natural remedy known to man. It's called urine therapy and consists of drinking one's own urine and rubbing one's entire body with it...*
>
> *The idea of drinking urine for medicinal purposes certainly takes some getting used to, but consider the facts about urine...*
>
> *'Urine therapy has been around for a long time...' said one NYC private practitioner who supports the therapy...When you have something that works, that's been around for a long time, even though it doesn't fit into any of the 'scientific' approaches, and there are many things that don't, I would say try it...if I had AIDS I would definitely try it.'"*

Ironically, urine therapy is one of the most scientifically corroborated of all natural therapies, and has been a scientific healing approach used for almost a century by mainstream medical researchers.

The article goes on to describe the case of one AIDS patient who reportedly had excellent results with urine therapy:

> *"Quique Palladino was diagnosed with AIDS, Kaposi's Sarcoma (a type of cancer common to AIDS patients), and numerous infections last year. Today, he claims to have gone into complete remission thanks to urine therapy. 'At first I just laughed and made jokes, he says...but they said that you could start by applying it topically...'*
>
> *'I had a terrible case of athlete's foot/ringworm that nothing seemed to work for. I started applying urine to it. After three days, the infection was completely gone. After that I was so convinced that I didn't mind drinking it.'*
>
> *'All my KS (cancer) lesions are [now] gone. The mouth ulcers that used to plague me have not returned. I used to have monthly outbreaks of genital herpes, but that's gone too. And even more importantly, my T-cell count has gone up.'"*

The article continues:

> *"More and more people are trying urine therapy now and they're reporting amazing results,' says Gene Ledorko, president of H.F.A. (Health, Education, AIDS Liaison), a group that meets weekly in New York City to discuss alternative and often holistic therapies for AIDS."*

There's also another extremely important recent medical discovery regarding urine and AIDS:

Bay Area Reporter
August 9, 1990

> *"Thanks to the research of Dr. Alvin Friedman-Kien and his staff at the New York University Medical Center it was discovered in 1988 **that the antibodies to HIV-1 appear in the urine of patients diagnosed with AIDS.***
>
> *...according to the involved researchers **'urine is not considered infectious because it has not been shown to contain the virus, only the antibodies'.** Blood often contains the HIV-1 and other potentially infectious agents such as hepatitis B.*
>
> *Urine is a 'sterile' fluid that is not found to contain viruses such as HIV-1 or hepatitis B except in individuals who may have an underlying kidney disease.'"*

A recent article in a doctors' journal that emphasizes natural medical treatments revealed that Dr. S. Burzynski, who discovered the naturally occurring anti-cancer urine proteins called antineoplastons, is now conducting FDA-approved research on the use of urinary antineoplastons in treating AIDS:

> *"According to Dr. Burzynski's research, antineoplastons are naturally occurring peptides and amino acid derivatives which are components of a biochemical defense system which parallels our immune system and protects us by reprogramming, or normalizing defective cells that may lead to disorders **such as cancer, AIDS, autoimmune diseases, benign tumors, etc."***
> **Townsend Letter For Doctors**
> **June, 1993**

During allergy research studies (see following section on allergies), in using natural urine therapy for allergy patients, it was also noted that urine:

"...greatly increased immune response, noticeably affecting and increasing the T-cell population and the body's resistance to viral infections."
Physician's Handbook on Immuno-Tolerance

This same research report also revealed that:

"There seems to be an enhanced response or stimulation of the immune system, mostly of the T-cell population [with the use of urine therapy]. While under treatment, patients reported an absence of viral diseases ('flu', colds, etc.), or greatly decreased symptoms.

On a few patients who exhibited low T-cell counts, the T-cell population was restored to normal after finishing their treatment..."

In the studies that have been presented so far, we've seen that many doctors and researchers using natural urine therapy have produced amazing cures for a wide variety of viral and bacterial illnesses, all of which is significant for AIDS patients.

There are also more testimonials and information on the treatment of AIDS with urine therapy in Chapters 6 and 7.

URINE THERAPY AND ALLERGIES

The field of allergy research is so huge and so complicated that the average person, let alone allergy researchers, find it difficult to understand it all. But one thing we do all know about allergies is that now almost everyone has one – or more.
Scientists don't really know for certain just what exactly is the mechanism in the body that is responsible for allergic reactions, but they do know that for some reason, an allergy sufferer's immune system begins to identify ordinarily harmless substances as harmful.

All of us know that our body produces white blood cells that search out and destroy harmful bacteria or viruses in the body, but in the case of most allergies, for some reason, the white blood cells attack substances that may be no threat to the body at all.

Like plant pollen, for instance. Pollen is a natural, vital substance in our environment which we normally breathe in with no problem. No problem, that is, for some people – but a big one for those whose immune systems identify it as a foreign and health-threatening substance; then the sneezing, sinus congestion and headaches, etc. of the "common" allergy attack begins.

We all eat foods like breads and grains because we know from centuries of experience that they're good for us. But in reality, more and more people today are discovering that foods that are great for everyone else produce often violent, negative reactions in their bodies.

So why does a person's immune system identify historically harmless substances as enemies? No one knows the answer to that, but what scientists do know is that when the immune system does identify a substance as a threatening foreign protein in the body, it sends out specific white blood cells (T and B lymphocytes) to attack it.

The "B" cells search out, identify and actually bind with the foreign protein (called an allergen or antigen), while the "T" cells rapidly divide, producing antibodies and large numbers of new T cells that will also be programmed to attack this antigen. Both the T and B cells actually have the ability to 'remember' this antigen, or foreign protein, and will attack it again when and if it reappears. In immunology, which is the study of immune system functions, this allergic response is referred to as the antigen-antibody conflict.

This is one reason why we have allergic reactions to the same substance over and over again – because our body has been programmed to attack even an ordinarily harmless substance, as though it's a threat to the body. This allergic reaction may sometimes be controlled by just eliminating the foods or cat hair, or soap, etc. that you're allergic to, but sometimes it's not that simple.

Sometimes it's impossible to avoid what we're allergic to and, even worse, a person's immune system can further malfunction and actually begin to attack the body's own internal cells, resulting in what are called autoimmune diseases such as lupus or rheumatoid arthritis. These auto-immune diseases are, of course, damaging to the body and in some cases can even be life-threatening.

Modern medicine has no cure for allergies and autoimmune diseases. And what is more disconcerting, allergies and related disorders are becoming more and more prevalent in our industrialized societies.

Researchers and doctors who deal with allergies, called immunologists, largely believe that allergies are essentially induced by unidentified weaknesses or alterations in the immune system. When the immune system is weakened or impaired, its ability to distinguish between harmless and harmful substances also becomes impaired. So your white blood cells, whose work it is to search out and destroy harmful proteins in the body, may begin to attack even ordinarily beneficial or benign proteins such as those that come from normal foods.

Immunologists also speculate that because our bodies are now exposed to enormous numbers of new chemical substances in our modern industrialized societies, that the immune system can become over-whelmed in its efforts to identify and deal with each new substance:

> *"It has been estimated that in the industrialized countries, man comes in contact with 150,000 man-made substances; pesticides, plastics, chemicals, etc., and that every year 5,000 new ones are manufactured. Is it any wonder then, that the immune system is hard-pressed to cope with this tremendous amount of 'foreign substances'?"*
>
> *It is all too possible that in the coming years, 100% of the population of the United States will suffer, to a lesser or greater degree, from some form of allergy or intolerance."*
> **Immuno-Tolerance Physician's Handbook, 1982**

Conventional doctors offer allergy sufferers decongestants, antihista-mines, anti-inflammatory drugs, immunosuppressants, etc., but the problem with these treatments is that they suppress or interfere with the optimal functioning of our immune systems, further weakening them and making us even more susceptible to disease and allergic reactions.

Many people with simple or severe allergies get extremely discouraged because they spend a fortune going from doctor to doctor without get-ting results. Not only do they not get rid of the allergic symptoms, but in many cases, they can't even find out what they're allergic to because our current diagnostic methods for allergies are crude and ineffective.

Identifying the specific antigen that a person is reacting to is a huge headache for doctors and their patients. And even if the allergy is iden-tified, there's still no effective conventional treatment for it.

This is where urine therapy comes in. Researchers have discovered that urine contains specific anti-allergen antibodies that are manufactured by the body itself and that when re-introduced back into the body through urine therapy, the allergic response is stopped.
Also, with urine therapy, there is less need to identify all the different things that you may be reacting to because the body will identify the allergens and will produce an antibody to correct the body's improper immune response that produced the allergy in the first place.

In extensive clinical testing with urine therapy on allergy patients, both in Europe and the U.S., allergy researchers and physicians noted incredible and often dramatic, rapid improvements, and also observed that urine is effective on an extremely wide range of food and chemical sensitivities. The following reports demonstrate the seriousness with which urine therapy has recently been utilized in the field of allergy treatment and research.

As medical researchers have discovered, allergic responses are caused by "renegade" white blood cells that inappropriately attack substances even when they may be no threat to the body. So it is the activity of these renegade white blood cells, called antigen receptors, that needs to be corrected in order to cure the allergy.

Report #32 **TITLE:** *SPECIFIC IMMUNOLOGIC UNRESPONSIVENESS,* 1982, by Dr. William D. Linscott, PhD, (published in Basic and Clinical Immunology).

Dr. Linscott's studies showed that when these antigen receptors (or renegade white blood cells), were re-introduced into the body, the body actually developed antibodies to these antigen receptors, and the antibodies then stopped the allergic response:

> *"These antigen receptors are found in low concentrations in urine. By injecting the receptors, it has been possible to induce antibody against the antigen receptors which can then limit or even abort an ongoing allergic response. These antibodies may in fact be an important regulator of the immune response."*

Linscott's study was one of the important works on which recent investigations into the use of urine in allergy treatments was based, because it gave allergists the clue as to how the body can be naturally stimulated to internally correct allergic reactions.

Realizing that the urine of allergic individuals contains the allergy-causing white blood cells, allergy researchers, as in the next report, reasoned that by giving allergic individuals their own urine internally, their bodies would develop antibodies to the renegade white blood cells contained in the urine which would then stop the allergic response. When urine therapy was administered during clinical allergy treatments, it produced excellent and often incredible results, as you'll see in the following reports.

This was an award-winning report delivered at the Oxford Medical Symposium in March, 1981, dealing with the treatment of allergies with urine therapy.

TITLE: *THE USE OF INJECTED AND SUBLINGUAL URINE IN THE TREATMENT OF ALLERGIES,* 1981, by Dr. Nancy Dunne.   *Report #33*

Dr. Nancy Dunne was medical advisor to the Irish Allergy Treatment and Research Association, founder of the Irish Orthomolecular Medical Association and a member of several allergy research societies:

"A simple technique for treating allergies – Auto-Immune Urine Therapy (A.I.U.) is rapidly gaining recognition in the United States and may well prove to be the method of the future. The rationale behind it is that by re-cycling the patient's urine, the protein globulins of which contain specific antibodies to allergens currently producing reactions, immunity from the antigen-antibody conflict (allergic reaction) is brought about.

I first learned of the method from Dr. William Fife (of California), while studying psychiatric developments in the U.S. in 1979. Dr. Fife, a neuropsychiatrist for 40 years had, some years previously, been forced to resign from his practice through ill health. Extensive investigations showed no disease. By chance he heard of A.I.U. therapy and following this treatment, enjoyed health and vigor he had not experienced for many years. He resumed full-time practice and now employs the same technique on his patients.

The main attraction of A.I.U. is that it eliminates the need to identify specific allergens – instead it makes use of the body's own identification system which is infallible for each individual. No sophisticated equipment is needed and the method, which is uncomplicated and safe, can be learned quickly. In addition, after treatment the patient is free to eat and drink without developing symptoms. These factors bring A.I.U. therapy within the reach of the average busy general practitioner who has not the time for detailed study of the varied diagnostic and therapeutic techniques used in this area of clinical ecology...

Injections are normally given once weekly. The number of treatments required to render a patient asymptomatic varies with the individual...In a series of clinical trials by Dr. Fife and his co-workers, A.I.U. therapy provided clinical relief lasting many years without further treatment in over 80% of cases. Statistics from his clinic show

92.6% of patients had more than 50% relief, while the average reported by patients themselves was 70%...

In the process of treating psychiatric patients, Dr. Fife found many apparent physical illnesses co-incidentally relieved, such as **multiple sclerosis, colitis, hypertension, lupus erythematosus, rheuma-toid arthritis, hepatitis, hyper-activity, pancreatic insufficiency, psoriasis and eczema, diabetes, herpes zoster, mononucleosis and so on...**

Serious adverse reactions to urine injection therapy are unknown—in over 100,000 treatments, Dr. Fife has not had one. Minor reactions are limited to occasional resurgence of familiar allergic symptoms or slight temporary malaise...

Shortly after my own experience, I modified the technique to treat a 5-year-old hyperactive asthmatic male...eczema which covered the entire skin surface was present from birth. His face and scalp exuded yellow fluid, his eyelids drooped permanently and his nails blackened and fell off.

Patches of secondary infection from scratching produced frequent bouts of fever and adenitis (an inflammatory condition of a lymph node or gland). He could not use his hands which were semi-closed crusted claws and his whole appearance was revolting. When kept in one position for any length of time he stiffened and was unable to walk.

He had constant earaches and fits of hysteria...Specialists, hospitaliza-tions and even forms of alternative medicine failed to give any relief. He was on regular antihistamines and sedatives and had many courses of antibiotics.

I instructed his mother to collect his midstream urine at the height of exacerbation of symptoms and, using an eye dropper, place 3 drops of urine under his tongue four times daily. The first time she used it he was having a screaming fit which usual-ly lasted half-an-hour – within one minute this subsided and he relaxed totally.

By the fourth day, there was noticeable discharge of viscous matter from the eczematous surface with the development of red spots everywhere. He also began each day sneezing and coughing with flowing mucous. His mother became alarmed at the copious discharge but was persuaded to persist, while at the same time tapering off all medication. By the sixth day the red spots changed to white, clear patches of skin were appearing, his eyelids no longer drooped and he was sleeping 4 hours *nightly at a stretch. After 2 weeks, he was off all medication, able to use his hands and walk freely, and no longer developed asthmatic attacks near grass or neighbor's pets.*

I increased his drops to six q.i.d. and he began to pass a much greater volume of urine daily with heavy whitish sediment. His hair darkened, healthy nails began developing and adults remarked on how placid he had become with his peers...two months later, his hyperactivity, hysteria, etc. were gone; he was sleeping soundly at night for the first time since birth — and apart from two small dry areas behind the knees, his skin was completely clear, and he was asymptomatic...

Auto-Immune Urine Therapy has much to offer compared to other allergy treatments. Tedious identification of all possible antigens (allergens) is not necessary. Equipment is minimal. Urine, being sterile, needs no preservatives. It is safe as [weakening] of the allergens] by the body eliminates the risk of anaphylactic shock...Drugs and chemicals — possible causes of side effects in sensitive patients — are not needed."

TITLE: *IMMUNO-TOLERANCE*, Physician's Handbook, 1982, from the International Immunology Institute, Canoga Park, California.

Report #34

This report is an extremely comprehensive and thoroughly detailed investigation into historical and current uses of urine therapy in treating allergies:

"The application, ingestion and injection of urine has been in existence for at least 4,000 years. It seemingly dies, only to reappear again, time after time. While other 'fad' or 'quack' treatments have disappeared, urine treatment has remained..."

The report goes on to mention several substantial clinical trials using urine therapy with excellent results. Researchers noted that urine injections not only provided a large measure of relief from allergic symptoms, but also seemed to boost the immune system:

"There seems to be an enhanced response or stimulation of the immune system, mostly of the T-cell population [with the use of urine therapy]. While under treatment, patients reported an absence of viral diseases ('flu', colds, etc.). or greatly decreased symptoms.

Young children, especially, seem resistant to colds (while under treatment), while their sisters and brothers (not receiving urine therapy) suffer from the usual repeated viral infections. Asthmatic patients with repeated sino-pulmonary infections report a remarkable decrease or absence of such repeated infections.

On a few patients who exhibited low T-cell counts, the T-cell population was restored to normal after finishing their treatment..."

This information is not only important for allergy sufferers, but, as mentioned, to AIDS patients as well, in that this disease is characterized by abnormally low T-cell counts that contribute to immune dysfunction.

Report #35

TITLE: *AUTO-IMMUNE THERAPY AGAINST HUMAN ALLERGIC DISEASE: A PHYSIOLOGICAL SELF DEFENCE FACTOR,* 1983, by C.W.M. Wilson and A. Lewis. Department of Geriatric Medicine, Law Hospital, Carluke, Scotland.

Wilson and Lewis, drawing on previous allergy research, and after their own extensive experimentation with the use of urine therapy in animals as a natural treatment for allergies, undertook the following research study on humans to determine the efficacy and correct dosage of urine in treating allergies.

Wilson and Lewis referred to urine therapy as Auto-Immune Buccal Urine Therapy (AIBUT). Buccal therapy is the oral administration of a medicine in which the substance is placed or held between the cheek and teeth or gums.

This research report stated that:

"It has been demonstrated that specific antibodies are secreted into the wall of the urinary tract. These findings indicate that allergens are secreted into the urine and that a subsequent antigen-antibody reaction is responsible for production of patients' allergic symptoms. In these circumstances it would be anticipated that administration of a patient's urine would prevent development of specific reactions caused by the range of allergens to which the patient is sensitive...

A pilot investigation has been carried out in twenty-five patients in order to discover an effective method of administration of urine, and to establish whether its therapeutic administration can alleviate allergic symptoms...

It was rapidly appreciated that undiluted urine was therapeutically effective for carrying out Auto-Immune Buccal Urine Therapy (AIBUT) in human beings.

AIBUT was initiated at times when it became obvious that the allergic condition had become uncontrollable, often in association with concurrent increased concentrations of extrinsic antigens in the air, such as pollens, molds, water particles in association with urban pollution, or increase in house dust or organic fumes associated with increase in central heating, house cleaning or painting...

AIBUT is performed by sub-lingual administration of pure urine. Use of diluted urine may produce incomplete symptom relief or actual potentiation of symptoms... The urine is obtained and administered prior to the principal meals against which it is providing protection...*

Symptoms from which the patient suffered prior to urine administration were noted.

The neutralizing dose is indicated when sensations of taste and temperature of the administered urine are no longer detected. The phenomenon of taste has been shown to be based on an immune reaction...

During the process of administration of AIBUT, allergic symptoms initially increase and then diminish as the sensation of taste and temperature alter and intensify and then disappear following repeated sublingual application of the urine drops...

The total number of drops administered constitutes the neutralizing dose. This dose should be administered before meals using urine collected since the preceding meal. The neutralizing dose is measured by the patient in terms of number of drops...It is administered with the aid of a mirror. The last 4 drops are administered separately in order to confirm by the absence of taste and temperature that the neutralizing dose is being taken.

[We conclude that] AIBUT is capable of controlling a wide range of food, extrinsic and chemical sensitivities."

After completing this clinical study, Wilson conducted additional research in 1984 on the use of urine in allergy treatment, and again concluded that it was an effective and highly desirable allergy treatment:

> *"The major advantage of AIBUT over other forms of anti-allergic therapy is that the allergic patient manufactures and uses his own urine for his own therapy...*
>
> *From a therapeutic aspect, AIBUT has advantages over other treatments such as dramatic restriction of allergenic foods, by food immunotherapy and by food neutralization.*
>
> *It is effective, it costs nothing and is easy to administer. The patient can be taught on the first occasion by the physician to recognize the neutralization end-point...The patient can then continue to administer AIBUT to himself, varying the dose as necessitated by changing food and environmental challenge."*

Wilson conducted additional experiments in order to determine the correct dosage of urine that would be therapeutically effective in both animal and human studies. He finally concluded that urine therapy for allergies should be administered by giving sublingual drops of urine until no taste or temperature was detected:

> *"The therapeutically effective dose of urine is determined as the point at which sublingual administration of urine drops cannot be detected by sensations of abnormal buccal (oral) taste or temperature by the patient when the drops are administered."*

In his study in 1984, Wilson also demonstrated that urine was effective as a treatment for the Raynaud Phenomenon, a condition which creates discoloration, coldness and sweating of the extremities, particularly the hands:

> *"Cold-water induced Raynaud symptoms were reduced in severity after administration of effective doses of unboiled urine in AIBUT."*

These reports on urine therapy and allergies are extraordinary indications of just how powerful and comprehensive urine therapy is and how may diverse health benefits it can offer, especially in view of the fact that so many of the illnesses we suffer from today are related to allergies.

MENTAL CONDITIONS

GENERAL RESEARCH INDICATIONS   *Report #36*

The effect of urine therapy on depression and other mental disorders such as hysteria, tantrums, etc. have been reported by many users of urine therapy including Drs. Dunne and Fife, the allergy specialists who were already mentioned:

> *"In the process of treating psychiatric patients, Dr. Fife found many apparent physical illnesses co-incidentally relieved, such as multiple sclerosis, colitis, hypertension, lupus erythematosus, rheumatoid arthritis, hepatitis, hyper-activity, pancreatic insufficiency, psoriasis and eczema, diabetes, herpes zoster, mononucleosis and so on...*
>
> **The reverse has also been noted by others who, in treating allergic physical illnesses find their patients' mental symptoms are concurrently abolished.***

I also have a newspaper clipping which reports that researchers have discovered that clinical depression may be caused by low levels of a brain chemical called PEA (phenylethylamine), which is a natural amphetamine-like substance that is constantly produced and broken down by the brain:

> **"Abnormally low amounts of PEA cause a lack of interest and concentration, loss of pleasure, forgetfulness, withdrawal from other people and other symptoms characteristic of depression.**
>
> **Researchers have learned that a key breakdown product of PEA, called PAA (phenyl acetate), is excreted in the urine in measurable amounts.***

PAA in urine may well play a part in the improvements in mental disorders that have been noted by users of urine therapy, although there are innumerable nutrients, therapeutic agents and undoubtedly other as yet unidentified elements in urine, such as hormones and other brain chemicals, that can also contribute to such improvements.

Report #37 **TITLE:** *BACTERICIDAL PROPERTIES OF URINE FOR NEISSERIA GONORRHOEAE* 1987 by Robert C. Noble, M.D. and M. Parekh, MS (From the Division of Infectious Disease, Department of Medicine, University of Kentucky College of Medicine). Published in the journal, Sexually Transmitted Diseases)

SUBJECT: EFFECT OF URINE ON GONORRHEA

This study was a follow-up to another research program (McCutcheon, et. al, 1977) that had investigated the gonorrhea bacteria-killing properties of urine and had reported that sufficiently concentrated urine can destroy the causative organism of gonorrhea and provide a natural immunity to the disease.

In 1987, Noble and Parekh confirmed McCutcheon's findings that concentrated urine could indeed kill gonorrhea bacteria:

> *"These results show that sufficiently concentrated, acidic urines kill gonorrhea bacteria by an unknown mechanism."*

Noble and Parekh also closely examined which constituents in the urine might be responsible for its anti-gonorrheal properties and concluded that increased acidity and concentration give urine its ability to destroy gonorrhea:

> *"Our study, like that of McCutcheon, et. al, found both the pH and the concentration of the urine to be important factors in the bactericidal activity of urine for gonococci."*

This research also demonstrated, as did Schlegel's, Cuellar's, O'Dell's and Kaye's, that elevated urea in urine was also capable of inhibiting gonorrhea bacterial growth:

> *"There was no growth of the gonorrhea bacteria after exposure to 100 mg of urea/ml."*

Again, oral urine therapy will increase urine acidity and urea concentrations in the system which in turn, as we've seen, can destroy a wide variety of disease organisms including gonorrhea.

We can also control and elevate urine acidity, if needed, through diet (*see Chapter 6 for information on how to do this and also how to monitor your urine pH levels at home*).

TITLE: *IDENTIFICATION OF A SPECIFIC INTERLEUKIN-1 INHIBITOR IN THE URINE OF FEBRILE PATIENTS*, 1984, by Zenghua Liao, et.al, published in the Journal of Experimental Medicine, Jan. 1984. (Dr. Liao was an exchange scholar from the Fujian Medical Center in China, and this study was supported by grants from the National Institutes of Health and others).

Report #38

Interleukin-1 (IL-1), among other things, is one of the body's immune defense substances which stimulates fever. Fever, as many of us know, helps the body destroy harmful microorganisms.

But researchers have discovered that not only does the body produce IL-1 during infection or attack, but that it also produces a substance that slows down, or suppresses the production of IL-1, presumably so that the body does not become too feverish or dangerously inflamed during the illness. This substance that keeps fever under control is called an IL-1 inhibitor.

Researchers discovered that this important IL-1 inhibitor substance was found not only in the blood, but in the urine also. In this study, the researchers found that the IL-1 inhibitor substance was present in both normal urine and the urine of febrile patients:

> *"These findings indicate that the IL-1 inhibitor is a normal constituent of human urine, but that the urine levels of this material are significantly increased in febrile states...* **We have found that the urine of febrile patients contains a potent IL-1 inhibitor.**
>
> **The urine of febrile patients has been found to contain high concentrations of IL-I,"**

Practitioners of urine therapy, including Duncan, Plesch, Armstrong, Wilson, Dunne and others have reported that internal urine therapy brings down fever during illness or inflammation during allergy attacks. This IL-1 inhibitor substance in urine may well play a part in urine's anti-inflammatory properties.

Report #39   **TITLE:** *UROKINASE, BASIC AND CLINICAL ASPECTS,* (book), 1982, by Dr. P.M. Mannucci and Dr. A. D'Angelo.

This book discusses several studies demonstrating the medical properties and applications of a urine ingredient called urokinase. In the studies, it was shown that urokinase could efficiently dissolve dangerous blood clots in the veins, arteries, heart and lungs that cause serious or fatal heart attacks, strokes etc. Urokinase was also shown effective in correcting ophthalmic (eyes) blood clots, bleeding, impaired circulation and in glaucoma therapy.

A drug form of urokinase, which has been called a "miracle blood clot dissolver", has been available for several years but isn't routinely used because it has been shown to cause serious side effects such as bleeding.

But for non-crisis care we don't need to take the drug and worry about side effects in order to get the benefits of urokinase because it's already naturally available in urine in measurable amounts and in safe concentrations. As this study revealed:

> *Urokinase exists in several molecular forms and can be found in freshly voided urine.*

> *A single chain, high molecular weight urokinase has recently been isolated from freshly voided urine. (1981, Husain, Garewich, and Lipinski).*

> *Urokinase can efficiently treat and even dissolve dangerous blood clots in the arteries and veins that can block blood vessels and lead to such conditions as strokes and heart attacks.*

This natural blood-clot dissolver in urine is certainly of tremendous significance and benefit in long-term preventive health care, and we can get the benefits of urokinase easily, without side effects, and at no cost when we use urine therapy regularly.

URINE THERAPY AND SKIN TREATMENTS
THE DERMATOLOGICAL AND COSMETIC APPLICATIONS OF URINE

The next three reports deal with current research on skin moisturizers and the use of urea as a moisturizer and skin treatment for various skin conditions including dry, scaling skin, eczema, rashes, etc.

Most of us have no idea that urea, which is the primary solid of urine, is a scientifically proven moisturizer, but as these studies reveal, urea is a far better moisturizer and skin treatment than even the most expensive oil-based creams or lotion that you can buy or get as a prescription from your doctor. Urine itself has long been used as an extremely effective treatment for skin diseases and dry skin conditions. These studies on urea demonstrate, in part, why urine is so successful in skin therapy.

TITLE: *UREA IN THE TREATMENT OF DRY SKIN*, 1992 by Dr. Gunnar Swanbeck, Department of Dermatology, Goteborg, Sweden.

Report #40

Unknown to most of us, urea has tremendous dermatological value as a skin moisturizer, and as treatment for eczema, psoriasis and other skin disorders. As Dr. Swanbeck states:

> *"Urea is a unique physiological substance. It has frequently been used in dermatological therapy for more than 20 years...*
>
> *Urea has been used extensively during the last two decades in the treatment of dry skin, both clinically and in cosmetic products. Its popularity is probably due to its effectiveness, good cosmetic properties and its being non-toxic and non-allergenic."*

Swanbeck goes on to say that skin needs water, not oils, to make it soft and younger looking. And urea naturally binds water in the horny layer of the skin, making it soft and pliable.

Almost all of the commercial and often astronomically expensive lotions and creams we buy to soften dry skin are composed of lipids, or oily substances, like mineral oil, which we think will moisturize and beautify our skin. But in reality, as Swanbeck points out, urea does a much better job of moisturizing the skin than oil-based moisturizers because it keeps water within the skin layers, making it supple and soft:

> *"Urea binds water in the horny layer. In 1952 Blank showed that the horny layer needs water – and not lipids – (oils) to become soft and pliable.*
>
> *In 1968 I showed that, when used on patients with psoriasis and severely dry skin, urea strongly increased the water binding capacity..."*

Ichthyosis is an inherited skin disorder in which the skin becomes extremely dry and fissured, resembling fish scales. Swanbeck and other researchers have found that urea is a safe and effective treatment even for this difficult-to-treat skin condition as well as for psoriasis and dry skin in general. Swanbeck continues:

> *"Urea has an antipruritic (anti-itching) effect that can be demonstrated experimentally in a controlled double-blind study...In diseases such as eczema this [anti-itching] property may be of importance.*
>
> *Urea has been shown to be clinically effective...A large number of studies have confirmed the beneficial effect of urea creams.*
>
> *Urea creams are useful for all degrees of dry skin. It was soon evident that urea creams were also useful for other dry skin conditions, even dry skin without any sign of diseases...There seems to be a self-regulating effect of urea creams. If the skin is very dry and scaly, a large amount of the cream is taken up by the horny layer. But if the horny layer is thin and has a normal water content, very little of the cream is actually taken up when the cream is applied in a normal way...Another disease where urea creams are of great value is hand eczema, especially the irritative and [allergic] type...*
>
> *Side effects of the use of urea creams: No long-term side effects have been found. To my knowledge, there is no report published of contact allergy. In spite of common use for many years, no epidermal or dermal atrophy (shrinking or wasting) has been reported with the use of urea."*

Swanbeck mentions that urea creams may have a stinging effect, especially on children, but other research confirmed that the urea stings only because it is absorbed so deeply into the skin layers and not because it is actually irritating or damaging to the skin. Urea creams are obviously effective on skin disorders, but whole urine is equally effective and safe, and usually does not sting on application which makes it easy to use. Instructions for use of urine in skin conditions are included in Chapter 6.

TITLE: *A THREE-HOUR TEST FOR RAPID COMPARISON OF EFFECTS OF MOISTURIZERS AND ACTIVE CONSTITUENTS (UREA),* 1992, by Jorgen Serup, M.D., Ph.D, Department of Dermatology, Bioengineering and Skin Research Laboratory, University of Copenhagen, Denmark. Published in Acta Derm Venereol, 1992.

Report #41

This is an interesting study which compares the effectiveness of five different types of urea creams to two other non-urea lotions, one of which is the well-known commercial skin moisturizer, Nivea. The results determined that urea creams were much better moisturizers than oil-based creams or lotions.

When ranked against Nivea and another lotion containing peanut oil, mineral oil, glycerin and a variety of other ingredients, the urea creams consistently outranked Nivea and the other oil-based lotion.

Actually, all the urea creams tested far outranked the well-known commercial, "doctor-recommended" Nivea cream. As a matter of fact, in this study, Nivea ranked last in moisturizing effectiveness – it was shown to be only slightly better than untreated skin!

Lotions containing even 3% urea ranked higher than Nivea, while the other oil-based lotion also showed a tendency to be much less efficient.

I've been in the hospital many times, and I've always been given Nivea or some other mineral oil-based lotion along with the other usual hospital amenities – but I've certainly never received urea lotions. Wouldn't it make a lot more sense for hospitals and health care providers to give out urea moisturizing lotions that have been medically proven to be best? And urea's extremely inexpensive – so why not use it? The next report provides some answers.

Report #42   TITLE: *INTRODUCTION TO A DOUBLE-BLIND COMPARISON OF TWO CREAMS CONTAINING UREA AS THE ACTIVE INGREDIENT,* 1992, by Dr. Jorgen Serup, University of Copenhagen, Denmark.

Dr. Serup undertook this study in order to determine what concentration of urea is needed in order to provide effective skin moisturizing. He begins this introduction to his report (see next page) with a short explanation for why urea's proven moisturizing properties have been generally ignored:

> *"The development of modern oil-based creams has created a silent revolution in dermatology.* **Today, the use of oils as moisturizers is a billion dollar business.**
>
> *However, dermatologists have shown only a limited interest in the scientific evaluation of the effects of oil-based creams and lotions on the skin, in that interest is now being directed more towards other revolutions in skin treatments such as topical corticosteroids (hormone creams) and retinoids."*

As Dr. Serup comments, scientists may know about the extraordinary moisturizing effects of urea, but cosmetic companies aren't interested in the scientific proof on urea because it isn't particularly glamorous, costs next to nothing and can't be patented, whereas different oil-based or chemical 'secret formulas' can be patented and glamorized.

> *"Scientific knowledge regarding moisturizers is concentrated mainly in the big international cosmetic companies which have to satisfy a world of dreams; also secrecy is a part of competition."*

But the fact that cosmetic companies can't make huge profits on urea creams doesn't change the fact that it's one of the best and least expensive skin treatments in the world – and you can get all of the benefits of urea simply by using urine on the skin (see Chapter 6).

Dr. Serup continues:

> *"Urea has a long history in dermatology, originally being used for the treatment of ulcers. Today it is used as a keratolytic (skin treatment) agent and as an active ingredient in moisturizing lotions for the treatment of ichthyosis (abnormal fissured, scaling skin), dry skin and various dermatitic conditions including atopy (intensely itchy skin inflammation). Urea is antipruritic (anti-itching), and antimicrobial...*

Interest in urea treatment declined in the 1970's, probably because many patients with atopic dermatitis complained of stinging sensations following the application of urea creams. This then was interpreted as being an irritant effect of urea on the skin. At that time, the documentation of urea was mainly clinical. Furthermore, research methods and knowledge about the effects of irritants on the skin had not yet attained their recently achieved labels.

Today, it is clear that stinging, resulting from 2%, 5% or 10% creams, is due to hyperosmolarity (intense penetration) of the creams, and is not a true irritant effect of the cytotoxic type.

It was Professor Gunnar Swanbeck who, in Scandinavia, introduced modern treatment with urea. In Germany, Professor W. Raab organized an international symposium in Salzburg...In Japan, Professor H. Tagami and his group have conducted a number of studies on urea and atopy (intensely itchy skin inflammations), presented at different meetings. Thus, interest in urea internationally is increasing, and it may be undergoing a renaissance within dermatology.

One can therefore see there are good reasons to revisit urea and to update our knowledge on this useful agent."

TITLE: *A DOUBLE-BLIND COMPARISON OF TWO CREAMS CONTAINING UREA AS THE ACTIVE INGREDIENT,* 1992, by Jorgen Serup, M.D., Ph.D, Department of Dermatology, Bioengineering and Skin Research Laboratory, University of Copenhagen, Denmark. Published in Acta Derm Venereol.

Report #43

Dr. Serup's report on the effectiveness of different urea concentrations in moisturizing creams begins with a short history of urea in dermatology:

"In medicine, urea was used for many years for a variety of conditions, including wound healing. As long ago as 1943, Rattner had used urea in hand creams as a humidity promoting additive...

Swanbeck, who studied urea treatment of ichthyosis, became the originator of the HTH urea-lactic acid cream, which is used extensively for a variety of keratotic (skin) conditions...

The many effects of urea on human skin were recently reviewed extensively...

The purpose of the present study was to evaluate the efficacy and toxicity of a 10% urea cream intended for dermatological treatment with a new 3% urea cream intended for cosmetological use...

"Blind" clinical evaluation by a dermatologist showed that 3% and 10% creams were equally and highly effective.

The reduction of dry skin, was the same in both treatment groups, but the 3% cream made the skin softer and more pliable, so the 3% cream was deemed cosmetically more acceptable.

No cases of skin irritation were reported.

In conclusion, the 3% and 10% urea creams were both found efficient, resulting in improvement of hydration and reduction of scaling. Both were non-toxic."

You could be presently using a commercial urea creams without even knowing it, so by way of information, these are a few urea creams that are mentioned in the Over-The Counter Physician's Desk Reference (PDR) drug guide:

- Aqua Care Cream (Menley & James)
- Aqua Care Lotion (Menley & James)
- Carmol 10 Lotion (Syntex)
- Eucerin Plus Moisturizing Lotion (Beiersdorf)
- Pen-Kera Creme (Ascher)
- Ultra Mide 25 Cream (Baker Cummins)

These are a few prescription urea creams also mentioned in the PDR:

AMINO-CERV: This cream is formulated for cervical treatments such as postpartum cervical tears and mild cervicitis (external female genital itching due to inflammation of the cervix).

ATTRAC-TAIN: Moisturizing Cream and Lotion; (this is a combination of urea and lactic acid which Swanbeck, Serup and others found to be very effective in treating even tough cases of intense itching and dry skin. Contains no petrolatum, mineral oil, parabens, dyes or perfumes).

UREACIN 10 LOTION, UREACIN 20 CREME, UREACIN 40 CREME: These three urea preparations contain 10, 20 and 40 % urea respectively, but again, the last study showed that you don't need such high urea concentrations to gain effectiveness, and concentrated urea can cause stinging, whereas natural urine usually does not.

Serup also discusses the fact that urea is much more than just a moisturizer because, unlike other creams and moisturizers, it has many different beneficial effects on the skin: it not only acts as an extraordinary therapeutic agent for skin disorders, but also attracts moisture to the skin while at the same time preventing water loss in the skin layers.

There is a completely all-natural urea lotion and cream formula now available called PureaSkin™. This preparation is excellent for reducing aging and water loss in the skin layers. The formula is available in both 10% and 20% urea concentrations. The 20% cream can be used for therapeutic purposes such as treating eczema, psoriasis, deeply cracked, dried or damaged skin, etc. The PureaSkin formulas contain no synthetic additives, preservatives or alcohol and are also hypo-allergenic.

Normal urine itself contains 2% urea and this percentage increases if you're using fresh urine internally. And as you've read, 3% urea is just as effective as higher urea concentrations in treating skin conditions, so your urine which is already 2% or more, will be an extremely effective skin treatment which can actually be combined with PureaSkin for added moisturizing and therapeutic effects.

TITLE: *5-YEAR TREATMENT OF THE CHRONIC SYNDROME OF INAPPROPRIATE SECRETION OF ADH WITH ORAL UREA,* 1993, by Dr. G. Decaux, et.al., Department of Internal Medicine, Erasme University Hospital, Belgium).

Report #44

Don't let the title of this report confuse you. ADH simply means anti-diuretic hormone and ADH is released by the pituitary gland in order to retain proper water levels within the body.

But in some disorders, too much ADH is released and as a result the body retains too much water, which can dangerously dilute the amount of sodium in the blood and can be just as health-threatening as having too little water in the system.
This condition of excessive water retention and lowered sodium content is called hyponatremia. When hypo-natremia is caused by the release of too much ADH, the condition is referred to as SIADH.

SIADH itself is usually caused by infections such as meningitis or pneumonia, but normally disappears once the infection is gone. However, some people develop chronic SIADH which, for some unknown reason, can persist for years.

This report describes the case of a woman with chronic SIADH who was treated with oral urea:

"A 63 year old woman was seen for treatment of hyponatremia. She was first treated successfully by severely limiting her water intake. But during the following year, she had many episodes of confusion and severe water retention.

Demeclocycline was then given, but had to be stopped after a few days because of severe stomach upset. The patient was then treated with oral urea. Each dose was dissolved in 100 ml water with 15 g antacid and taken during or after a meal. She was asked not to drink more than 1500 ml/day. During the following year she never presented symptoms of excess water retention and she never complained of any side effects. At one point, doctors tried to replace the urea by a high salt supplementation but she complained of leg edema and developed stomach discomfort. The patient preferred to return to her oral urea therapy.

The patient was treated for 5 years with oral urea and has never again had symptoms related to water retention even though she is drinking a normal amount of fluids.

The treatment of this patient is the longest experience these researchers have had in administering urea for the treatment of hyponatremia – and this without any side effects."

As we've seen in many other studies, urine or urea has long been known to be an effective diuretic agent – and unlike synthetic prescription or commercial diuretics, can safely relieve excess water retention in the body.

CHAPTER SUMMARY

There are many other research studies related to the medical implications and uses of urine and urea which have not been mentioned in this chapter, but the selected reports that were presented do provide an overwhelmingly convincing and clear overview of the enormous medicinal value of urine therapy.

It seems unfortunate that these extraordinary research studies which have taken place over the course of nearly 100 years have been given no public attention, considering the suffering and deaths that might well have been prevented by the use of this most simple and inexpensive medicine, that even many doctors themselves admit can be used with great advantage by patients themselves at home.

As far as the use of urine extracts is concerned, as these studies show, natural urine extracts, such as those used in cancer treatments, obviously are of value and have been shown to stimulate remarkable healing. But as the research also demonstrates, there are a huge variety of elements in urine that have tremendous medicinal value, so using only one element or extract, and eliminating the rest has obvious drawbacks. Whole urine itself is obviously of immense importance in supporting the immune system and in delivering the maximum number of medicinal urine ingredients to the body.

But in treating tough diseases like AIDS, or cancer, for instance, the **combination** of urine extracts such as urea, antineo-plastons, HUD (Human Urine Derivative), etc., with whole urine therapy could play a vital role in healing difficult, advanced and intractable forms of disease by providing additional amounts of important medicinal urine elements to the system during times of intense illness.

This is not to say that difficult diseases have not been cured by natural urine therapy alone, they have, but in the case of AIDS, for example, supplementing natural urine therapy with oral or injected urea, in order to deliver an added concentration of urea and its anti-viral effect to the body could constitute an extremely effective treatment regimen.

Concentrated urea itself has been shown to completely dissolve viruses (McKay and Schroeder, 1935); its anti-bacterial and anti-fungal properties can prevent and heal infections, and it has been proven that even very high dosages of urea are safe and non-toxic (see pgs. 99-103). So it makes sense that urea supplementation, by raising the concentration of urea in the system, could be of great value in treating AIDS.

Researchers and doctors, however, by using urine extracts alone in many of these research studies, logically speaking, limited the impact of their treatments by eliminating the huge range of medicinal elements that whole urine offers. There is no apparent advantage to eliminating the concurrent use of whole urine with urine extracts, especially in view of the fact that natural urine, even in large quantities, has been shown to be safe and non-toxic. Hopefully, doctors, researchers and the medical community will recognize and begin to research and utilize this combined medical approach in the future.

Some in the conventional medical community may argue that although natural urine has been proven to contain an enormous variety of medicinally beneficial elements, that only concentrated urine extracts can give results because simply ingesting whole urine internally does not provide a strong enough concentration of these elements to produce appreciable beneficial results.

But as the clinical research studies show, ingestion and injection of natural urine and natural urine extracts does produce remarkable results. Also, as many of these studies demonstrate, the beneficial ingredients in urine are effective even though they may not be chemically concentrated:

1) The Japanese study in 1965 on the anti-TB elements in urine, stated that laboratory tests prove that *"these [anti-tubercule] substances [in urine] have so strong an activity that a very high dilution of them can inhibit the growth of tubercule bacilli..."*

In other words, even though these anti-TB elements in natural urine are unconcentrated and diluted, they are still extremely active and effective in stopping the growth of TB bacteria. This indicates that in using natural urine therapy, we can still get the benefit of strong anti-TB elements, even though they have not been chemically concentrated in drug or extract form.

2) The research studies showed that stronger concentrations of urea are anti-bacterial and anti-viral, and that we can increase the concentration of urea in our bodies by taking more urea. As one study stated, "Urine collected from volunteers after ingestion of urea demonstrated a marked increase in anti-bacterial activity, as compared with urine collected before ingestion of urea."
(Dr. D. Kaye, Anti-Bacterial Activity of Human Urine, 1968).

Because urine itself contains urea, we can increase the concentration of urea and its anti-bacterial activity in our systems through urine ingestion, as this study demonstrated.

3) Another study stated that: *"It is known, however, that the presence of antibody, **even in amounts which are not detectable by conventional methods, may prevent disease."** (Dr. Martin Lerner, Neutralizing Antibody to Polioviruses in Normal Human Urine, 1962).*

So even though the natural antibodies in your urine may be extremely minute and undetectable, these antibodies can, nevertheless, be effective in fighting and preventing diseases. And when we use oral urine therapy, we can get the benefits of these natural antibodies in low, safe concentrations, rather than as highly concentrated drug substances which overwhelm our natural immune defenses.

4) *Research on the use of natural urine therapy for allergies has repeatedly demonstrated the effectiveness of recycling individual natural urine antibodies:*

> *"A simple technique for treating allergies – Auto Immune Urine Therapy (A.I.U.) is rapidly gaining recognition in the United States and may well prove to be the method of the future. The rationale behind it is that by re-cycling the patient's urine, the protein globules of which contain specific antibodies to allergens currently producing reaction, immunity from antigen-antibody conflict is brought about...*
> ***Auto-Immune Urine Therapy has much to offer compared to other allergy treatments.*** *Tedious identification of all possible antigens (allergens) is not necessary. Equipment is minimal. Urine, being sterile, needs no preservatives.* ***It is safe as [weakening] of the allergens by the body eliminates the risk of anaphylactic shock...Drugs and chemicals – possible causes of side effects in sensitive patients – are not needed.***
> **(Dr. N.P. Dunne, The Use of Injected and Sublingual Urine in the Treatment of Allergies, 1981).**

As extensive research in many different fields of medicine has demonstrated, natural urine therapy is remarkably effective, and the fact that its constituents are in dilute concentrations can actually be considered an advantage in that they gently and safely stimulate the immune system.

Dr. Duncan and her colleague Dr. Fife reported that over 100,000 allergy patients were successfully treated with oral and injected natural urine therapy. Drs. Duncan, Plesch, Krebs, Wilson, Lewis, Garotescu, Tiberi and many other researchers have shown the extraordinary results that the use of an individual's own natural urine and urine constituents can produce on a wide variety of disorders.

As the researchers themselves comment, urine or urea therapy is such a remarkably safe, simple, and effective medicine that it richly deserves the full attention of the medical community and the public. And this is especially true today, as humanity searches for safer, saner methods of caring for and preserving our all-important health.

As a final conclusion to our review of the research and clinical studies, I'd like to finish up with an excellent summary on the medical use of urine therapy by Dr. Kurt Herz, a German obstetrician who successfully used the therapy in his practice and did much to promote the widespread use of it in Europe in the 1940's. In 1964, at the age of 84, Dr. Herz published an article in a German medical publication entitled "Autogenous Urine Therapy, Present and Future Prospects", which revealed many unknown facts about the history of urine therapy in

20th century medical practice, why it was discontinued and why it deserves to be resurrected and given public attention today:

"The history of medicine shows that whenever new therapies are introduced, established therapies are put aside and forgotten. In our age of 'miracle medicine' such a change is more obvious than ever. However, physicians frequently come to realize after many years that the positive results expected from the new therapies have not been achieved. At that point, we may reach out to new therapies or remorsefully fall back on those therapeutic modalities which were applied successfully in the past when all else failed.

Autogenous Urine Therapy (AUT) has been practiced for about 2000 years which makes it easy to understand why physicians and scientists throughout the ages have tried to uncover the secret behind it. I have practiced AUT since the early 1920's and in addition to successfully treating abnormalities in pregnancy, I was able to prove that pertussis (whooping cough) in its spastic phase could only be treated with the patient's whole urine, whereas fractions of it or urine of siblings showed no effect.

After treating several hundred patients, I presented my first publication on AUT in 1931. Since that time, hospitals and physicians from all branches of medicine have employed AUT and the list of indications for its use were expanded. AUT was, however, gradually forgotten due to the political upheavals of WW II. It is therefore not surprising that Dr. J. Plesch (London) erroneously portrayed AUT as a novelty in medicine in his publication in 1947, "Therapy with Urine." I replied to Plesch's work by publishing another article on AUT in a German medical journal 1947 in which I listed all the numerous doctors who were already successfully implementing urine therapy in their practices prior to Plesch in different forms and for varied symptoms. As a result of this article, a publishing company approached me and requested that I write a book on the subject, which I did.

My book was published in 1950, with a second edition in 1959. Since that time, interest in Auto Urine Therapy is again on the rise. Letters from Germany testify that physicians who have successfully tried this therapy want to continue it. Because of the advances in the diagnosis of viral infections, these diseases were primarily targeted for this therapy and fast and enduring positive results have been published...This therapeutic modality is presently being implemented differently in different countries. The fact that a book on urine therapy is presently being translated into French demonstrates that there is still as much interest in it now as there was during its early phase..."
Dr. Kurt Herz, M.D. (published in the German medical journal, Der Landartz, May 10, 1964.)

CHAPTER 5

THE HISTORY OF THE WORLD'S OLDEST MEDICINE

From earliest times, man has been curious about urine. Prior to the development of any written language, when signs were used to denote certain important materials or substances, it is interesting to note that urine was one of the substances identified with a specific sign. Below is the ancient symbol for urine, suggesting that it was recognized as one of the basic substances, or elements, of nature:

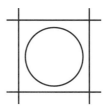

As many doctors and researchers in the twentieth century have noted, the medicinal use of urine does have an extremely long, varied and fascinating history:

> *"Of interest to us is the use of urine in primitive medicine, for there is scarcely a disease that has not been treated with it, either by external application or internal administration."*
> **Dr. H. Smith**
> **Journal of the American Medical Association**
> **July, 1954**

In the 17th century, the great pioneer in chemistry, Robert Doyle stated that:

> *"The virtues of human urine, as a medicine, would require an entire volume for their enumeration."*

As another doctor recently commented:

> *"Autouropathy (urine therapy) did flourish in many parts of the world and it continues to flourish today...there is, unknown to most of us, a*

wide usage of uropathy and a great volume of knowledge available showing the multitudinous advantages of this modality..."
Dr. J. Herman
Albert Einstein College of Medicine, N.Y., 1980

Let's take a closer look at just how people around the world, in almost every civilization, have used urine to heal themselves – long before science had proven it to be of extraordinary medical value.

The World's Oldest Medicine

Because the medicinal use of urine dates back even to the earliest civilizations, it's often been referred to as the world's oldest medicine:

EGYPT   One of the earliest therapeutic uses of urine has been traced to early Egyptian papyri. Medical papyri reportedly attest to the immense therapeutic value of both drinking and washing with urine in order to cure skin conditions.

ROME: The Roman writer and historian Pliny recounted many different therapeutic applications of urine. And, in addition to its medical use, urine was valuable in other ways to Roman and other ancient civilizations, because of its cleansing and softening properties. As reported in modern times, *"Urine is a weak detergent by virtue of its urea content and this detergent property is greatly enhanced when it is allowed to undergo bacterial fermentation, in consequence of which most or all of the urea is decomposed into the ammonium carbonate, a moderately alkaline salt. Such fermented urine has probably been used since time immemorial as a soap."*
Journal of the A.M.A., 1954

The modern urine therapist John Armstrong highly recommended the use of old urine in treating various types of wounds, especially those where deteriorated or decaying tissue were present. He observed that this "detergent" property of old urine was tremendously effective in cleansing wounds and promoting the growth of new tissue.

CHINA   In the book entitled Chinese Folk Medicine and Acupuncture,(1974), the author discusses the ancient practice of using 'human medicines' in China:

Along with herbs and plants, the Chinese esteemed a number of other pharmaceuticals, some of which were substances of the body. Most of them seem like unappetizing concoctions. But before we deride them as nonsense, let us not forget that during the recent World Wars I and II, urine was used in cases of emergency. Soldiers would apply the urine to their wounds as a disinfectant and healing agent – the urine of a healthy person is completely free of germs!

The treatment of slow-healing wounds with urea (the soluble nitrogenous substance of urine) often produces excellent results and is employed within the field of scientific medicine. A related example may be the traditional Chinese use of boys' urine in the treatment of pulmonary tuberculosis, a domestic remedy that is kept alive stubbornly in the folk-medicines even of Western countries. Swallowed warm, urine is said to remove hoarseness and soothe inflamed throats. Also very popular as a tonic and as a solvent for clogged blood vessels in pregnant women. It is to be taken three times a day, warm, mixed with a dash of wine."

INDIA

Urine therapy has an extremely lengthy and involved history in India, although as a whole, urine therapy was blended into the religious beliefs and practices of the country.

The earliest references to the medicinal use of urine in India are found in a 5000 year old religious Sanskrit text called the Damar Tantra, which contains 107 verses extolling the virtues of urine as a medicament, complete with extremely detailed instructions on everyday use. The Damar Tantra refers to urine therapy as Shivambu Kalp Viddhi, or Shivambu Kalpa, roughly translated, the "water of Shiva", (the god Shiva is the great destroyer and regenerator, and creator of the healing Ganges river). These verses make extremely interesting historical reading:

Verses 1-4: Oh Parvati! (the god Shiva speaking to his wife Parvati). The urine is to be drunk from pots made of Gold, Silver, Copper, Brass...Glass or Earth. The urine should be collected in any one of these utensils and should be drunk.

Verse 5: The follower of the therapy should avoid pungent, salty things in his meals. He should not over-exercise himself and should take balanced and light diet. He should sleep on the ground and control the senses.

Verse 7: The first and concluding flow of the urine is to be left out and the intermediate flow of urine is to be taken. This is the best process.

Verse 9: *Urine is a divine nectar! It is capable of abolishing Old Age and various types of diseases and ailments.*

Verse 28: *The extract of Mica and Sulphur should be dissolved in urine and taken regularly. It relieves the ailment of Dropsy (edema) and Rheumatism.*

Verse 36: *Rock Salt and Honey taken in equal proportions should be taken first in the early morning and it should be followed by urine. This makes man lustrous.*

Verse 40: *He who drinks the mixture of urine, honey and sugar is relieved of any type of ailment within a period of six months. His brain power becomes brilliant and his voice becomes melodious.*

Verse 45: *The urine should be boiled in an earthen pot and extracted to one-fourth quantity. It should then be allowed to cool. This extract then is used for the body massage.*

Verse 107: *Oh my beloved Parvati! I have narrated the details of urine therapy. This, then, is it's technique. Attempts should be made to keep it a secret. Do not tell anyone.*

Whatever Shiva's reasons for keeping it a secret, urine therapy did apparently work its way into the traditional system of Ayurvedic medicine for some time in India, and was generally used with herbal preparations for several centuries.

However, as a recent Indian author, Raojibhai Patel tells us, in his book, *Manav Mootra, (Auto-Urine Therapy)*, written in 1963:

> *"In the course of time, it appears that urine (as a natural medicine) was discarded...and the place of urine was taken up by purely herbal preparations. Allopathy (the use of synthetic drugs, surgery, etc.) is so advanced today and it has dominated the society to such an extent that Ayurveda (natural healing)... has been forgotten.*
>
> *The question naturally arises as to why urine, so valuable for health, has been given up in the present age. The only answer to this is that our views regarding the values of life have altered. We have moved away from Nature and have forgotten the use of natural means.*
>
> *Still, however, there are a number of men who like to be benefitted by this gift of nature. Lamas in Tibet have been freely using urine and...they have been able to keep their bodies healthy for a hundred and fifty years or even longer.*

The late Sir Morris Wilson had come to know of its use by Lamas, before his making his expedition to the highest peak of the Himalayas – Mt. Everest. While climbing, he had been drinking urine and was also rubbing it on the body."

There are several extremely enthusiastic advocates of urine therapy in India today who vigorously support a public revival of this age-old medicine.

Because it is a self-administered therapy requiring no medical intervention or fees, many prominent people in India, most notably, the former prime minister, Moraji Desai, see urine therapy as the perfect medical solution for the millions of Indians who cannot afford medical treatment.

Several fairly recent books and numerous magazine and newspaper articles have been devoted to the subject of urine therapy in India. Mr. Desai was even interviewed in 1978 on American television during the CBS news program "60 Minutes", during which he discussed the remarkable value of urine therapy at length with a surprised and skeptical Dan Rather.

Mr. Desai was unaware of the scientific data supporting the use of urine in medicine at the time of the interview, so his testimony almost totally lacked impact – but his courage, sincerity and concern were apparent. Incidentally, Mr. Desai was reportedly a healthy and vigorous 92 years of age in 1988, and still going strong.

ENGLAND

The earliest references to urine therapy in England are found in a curious book entitled *Salmon's English Physician, or the Druggist's Shop Open'd*, written in 1693 and dedicated to Queen Mary II by a Dr. Salmon, a 17th-century London "Professor of Physick". Salmon enthusiastically expostulates his views on the many uses and benefits of urine as a medicine:

"Urine is taken from Humane Kind, and most four-footed animals; but the former is that which is chiefly used in Physick and Chemistry. It is the Serum, or watery part of the Blood, which being directed by the emulgent Arteries to the Reins is there separated, and by the ferment of the parts, converted into urine. The urine. Drank it cures the hottest burning Fever and expels the malignity of the Disease, it provokes Urine, is good against the Dropsie (edema) and Jaundice, and dropt into the ears, helps Pain and Deafness in them; it is said also to heal Ulcers in the Mouth. Man or woman's urine is hot, dry, dissolving,

cleansing, resists Putrefaction; used inwardly against Obstructions of Liver, Spleen, Gall; as also against the Dropsie, Jaundice, Stoppage of the Terms in Women, the Plague, and all manner of malign Fevers."

The Indian book on urine therapy, *Manav Mootra*, originally published in 1963, also makes several references to historical English treatises on the medical uses of urine:

"The English physician Alis Barker holds that (urine) contains all the elements which destroy the poisonous germs of the body. Doctor T. Wilson Dichmann, a well-known physician of England writes in a journal that the 'composition of urine varies with every patient according to his bodily condition. Urine is the best remedy to cure all the diseases except the structural breakdown or deformity...Urine saves the doctor from the likely mistake in the selection of appropriate medicine...'

Ciril Scott in his book, Doctor, Diseases and Health, has given a beautiful description of the Urine Therapy practiced by the late W.H. Buxtor of Harrogate city, Leads, England in the following words: 'Mr. Buxtor used to drink his urine regularly. He had also written a number of articles on the uses of urine. He lived a long life, got rid of his pernicious cancer by applying urine packs and by drinking it...he held that drinking of urine is not only harmless but is positively useful.

Nowadays urine is being utilized in the preparation of cosmetics also. The chemists of England have prepared the best types of bathing soaps and quality creams from it. It means that the application of human urine had already been in vogue of which we were unaware."

FRANCE   The noted 19th century French chemist, Fourcroy in his extensive publications, devoted an entire volume to the composition of urine and wrote that:

"The urine of man is one of the animal matters that have been the most examined by chemists, and of which the examination has at the same time furnished the most singular discoveries to chemistry, and the most useful application to physiology, as well as the art of healing."

Wealthy French women of the 17th century reportedly took urine baths to beautify their skin. In the French treatise, Histoire de L'Academie Royale des Sciences, written in 1708 by M. Lemery urine is tastefully referred to as the "water of a thousand flowers". Lemery reports that it helped him to control and cure jaundice, rheumatism, gout, dropsy, vapors, sciatica and asthma. Eighteenth-century French dentists also reportedly used urine for curing various dental problems.

Americans have been using urine therapy for more than a hundred years. An article on the historical uses of urine therapy entitled Autourotherapy, by John R. Herman, M.D. appeared in June 1980 in the New York State Journal of Medicine. Herman gives an extremely thorough overview of early applications of urine therapy around the world and in America:

AMERICA

> *"Americans, too, utilized urine medically in the early days of medicine. In the archives of the Philadelphia Academy of Medicine is a letter from a Dr. Richard Hazeltine, M.D., of Maine, dated October, 1810, and entitled "Observations on the medical use of Human urine."*

Dr. Hazeltine wrote:

> *"From considering the most obvious qualities of urine, even a superficial observer would unhesitatingly conclude, that it is a substance possessed of no inconsiderable power, whether taken into the stomach; applied to the surface of the body; or injected into the body; and when its proximate principles are ascertained by the aid of chemical agents, one would feel himself warranted to place it among those articles which are capable of producing very evident effects on the living system...*

> *Ever since I can remember, I have been acquainted with the occasional internal use of urine as a domestic medicine, and my preceptor sometimes prescribed it...in the quantity of half an ounce to an ounce, sweetened with molasses to infants...Often in the age of childhood, after I had gone to bed, have I sip'd, and with no great reluctance, the steeming, salutiferous "buttered-flip"; administered by the careful hand of (many) an affectionate mother to her tender offspring who were affected with various catarrhal complaints, brought on by wet feet, and exposure to sudden vicissitudes of the weather.*

> *The 'buttered-flip' was composed of recent urine, obtained from one of the children, hot water, honey and a little butter; and it generally removed the complaints for which it was given.*

> *A very respectable elderly lady of the society of Friends, who formerly lived in Lynn, Massachusetts, and who justly acquired a high reputation and no inconsiderable authority as a nurse, has told me that urine was frequently exhibited in the same manner; she had thought proper to*

dignify the mixture of urine and molasses with the name of 'Salem flip'".

Dr. Herman who quoted this article asks both the medical community and the public to examine why there is such an undeserved historical prejudice against urine therapy:

"As mentioned before to most of the civilized peoples of the world there is a strange repugnance about drinking urine, even their own. Why this should be is questionable and the question is not answered by saying, 'It is a waste matter discarded from the body!'

Over most of the civilized world, blood and blood derivatives are used medicinally with no thought of the distaste usually associated with urotherapy. We utilize packed cells, plasma, white cells and various other fractions of the blood without pause.

Urine, too, is only a derivative of the blood. It contains, in its fresh condition, only those chemicals and compounds of the blood in circulation in each of us. If it is not toxic, or disgusting while in the blood, why does it suddenly become so abhorrent in the urine?

If the blood should not be considered unclean, then the urine also should not be so considered. It is only a derivative of the blood."

CONCLUSION

As we've seen in this and the preceding chapters, there is a great and almost overwhelming abundance of scientific, anecdotal and historical evidence supporting the efficacy of urine therapy.

The weight and strength of the scientific and anecdotal evidence clearly demonstrates the tremendous significance of this most maligned and yet most comprehensive and effective of natural medicines.

In this era of spiraling illness, drug-related deaths and exorbitant health care costs, natural urine therapy presents a proven medical treatment that must be taken out of the laboratory and given the full public attention and use that it deserves and has so rightly earned. None of us can afford to ignore the implications that the extraordinary curative powers of urine therapy hold for all of us – including our doctors.

Each of us has the primary responsibility to care for and maintain our own individual health, and urine therapy gives us an incomparable medical tool to heal our illnesses and to protect ourselves from disease.

And we don't have to travel anywhere or empty our bank accounts to get access to this miracle medicine – all we have to do is use it. Hopefully, we'll all have the wisdom to take full advantage of the magnificent benefits of this truly remarkable, freely-given and precious gift of nature.

CHAPTER 6

HOW TO USE THE THERAPY AT HOME

There are actually several ways to approach urine therapy. But before you begin, make sure you've read over the research studies in Chapter 4 that are pertinent to your condition and the information in this chapter first so that you can fully assess how to get the greatest benefit from the therapy. Also you may find that you want to use different methods at different times to deal with changing health conditions.

Getting Started

Before you start using the therapy, review your diet and general health habits. For best results with any health therapy, you need to be well-rested and be eating nutritious food.

For general help with improving your nutrition, the books listed below provide excellent information, and will give you the direction and guidance you may need to improve your diet:

Thirty Days to Better Nutrition
by Virginia Aronson
Easy but effective diet changes that can improve your health.

The McDougall Program
by Dr. John McDougal
A simple, effective 12-day dietary adjustment program for better health.

Food and Healing
by Annemarie Colbin
Learn how nutrition affects your health and how to use foods to help you heal.

If you are consistently overtired and your diet is full of refined sugar, processed foods, additives, chemicals, caffeine, soda, too much meat, over-the counter-drugs, etc., your body and immune defenses are not going to be able to function properly, and your ability to heal any disorder, large or small, will be impaired, no matter what medical treatment you use.

It's also important to realize that drug-taking and poor dietary habits impact on the quality of your urine; the more good nutrients you put into your body, the more effective urine therapy will be for you.

Your urine is a direct reflection of what you're taking into your body, so it only makes sense that recycling quality nutrients during urine therapy is going to give better results than recirculating synthetic additives, preservatives, refined, de-natured flours, sugars, caffeine, nicotine, etc.

Keeping a daily health journal.

Keeping a daily health journal is also an excellent practice while using urine therapy – it can help you tremendously to become familiar with your reactions to different foods and substances and to learn your body's patterns, such as blood pressure, acid levels, sugar levels, etc., so that you can more easily detect and correct abnormalities that can be precursors to or indications of illness or disease.

These are the basic forms of urine therapy that can be used at home:

INTERNAL USE:

1. Oral Drops
2. 1-4 oz. quantities
3. Fasting on large quantities
4. Homeopathic urine or urea
5. Urea Crystals (See Order Form in back of book)

EXTERNAL USE:

1. Skin Massages
2. Compresses and packs
3. Foot or full baths
4. Ear, nose and eye drops
5. Enemas
6. Urea Crystals (for wound healing, external ulcers, etc.)

The following are general instructions on using these methods of urine therapy at home which are based on the research reports and people's personal experiences, but as you become familiar with the different methods, you'll find that you develop your own techniques.

Remember that these instructions are not given as medical advice, but are simply to be considered as general information which is contained in the research studies or has been retold in anecdotal accounts.

GENERAL INSTRUCTIONS

INTERNAL USE

1. COLLECT MIDSTREAM URINE IN A CLEAN CUP OR CONTAINER

A clean glass or clear plastic container is best for collecting the urine. In the research studies, urine is usually collected by means of a "clean catch" in which the genital area is cleansed before collecting the urine. This is important for women in particular when using urine therapy internally and can be done by simply washing with a little soap and water. Collect the midstream urine only.

You can take along pre-packaged clean catch kits which include a sterile cup and antiseptic paper towelettes for convenience during travel or whenever unsanitary living conditions or contaminated water are a problem.

2. ALWAYS USE FRESH URINE IMMEDIATELY UPON COLLECTION

Urine breaks down quickly outside the body so use it internally as soon as you collect it. If you are going to use it for external use only, this isn't as important, as you can use either fresh or old urine for most external applications.

3. BEGIN WITH ORAL DROPS THEN INCREASE DOSAGE AS NEEDED

Once you've read the book and are ready to begin using the therapy, **START BY TAKING A ONLY FEW DROPS EACH DAY IN ORDER TO LET YOUR BODY ADJUST GRADUALLY.**

Fill a clean medicine dropper from the cup of urine and place one or two drops under your tongue. This method lets you get used to the taste slowly and will still give you health benefits. You can slowly increase and adjust the amount later when you've determined what amount is right for your condition.

    1). Start by taking 1-5 drops of morning urine on the first day.

    2). The second day, take 5-10 drops in the morning.

3). On the third day, take 5-10 drops in the morning, and the same amount in the evening before you go to bed.

4). Once you feel accustomed to the therapy, gradually increase the amount as needed for obtaining results for your condition. As you use the therapy, you will learn to adjust the amount you need by observing your reactions to the therapy. More information on dosage is given further on in this chapter.

4. DO NOT BOIL OR DILUTE THE URINE

Research studies show that boiling urine destroys many of its medicinal properties, so when taking it internally, use it only in its fresh, natural form. Research studies have also shown that diluting urine (or urea) decreases its antibacterial activity, so rather than diluting it in juice or water to get accustomed to using it, use a few oral drops instead.

5. HOMEOPATHIC URINE

The importance of using urine collected at the beginning or height of acute symptoms of illness, particularly infections and allergies, has been suggested by some researchers, because this urine contains the greatest amount of antibodies and immune-defense agents with which the body is already fighting the illness. A homeopathic preparation preserves this potent first-stage-illness urine and can then be used throughout the duration of the illness.

Homeopathic urine is also excellent for children. For those of you with extreme sensitivity or toxicity, who may feel that you are getting too strong a reaction to the urine initially, try using it as a homeopathic dilution. Instructions on how to prepare a diluted, but very effective form of urine are included in the section, Homeopathy and Urine Therapy, further on in this chapter.

6. MONITOR AND BALANCE YOUR PH

pH refers to the acid/alkaline condition of the body. The body is normally mildly acidic, and maintaining the proper pH is crucial in urine therapy. pH values naturally change throughout the day. **Morning urine is generally more acidic than mid-day urine, and pH also changes in response to diet** – in general, foods like meats, coffee, alcohol, milk, eggs and beans make the body more acidic while most fruits and vegetables have an alkaline effect. (See Appendix for a more complete listing of acid/alkaline foods).

It's always good to keep an eye on both your urine and saliva pH levels, because both should present a proper acid/alkaline balance.

The ideal pH range of saliva is about 6.4 - 7.2, (below 6.4 is too acidic, above 7.2 is too alkaline). Saliva usually becomes more alkaline after eating and with a vegetarian diet.

Urine pH should ideally vary from approximately 5.0 (acid in the morning) to 8.0 (alkaline at night) during each 24-hour period.

If your urine or saliva pH levels are consistently out of range for a long period of time, it means that your body is not functioning correctly or that your diet is consistently too acid or too alkaline.

pH measuring strips with numerical values are commercially available for testing your acid/alkaline levels and make it simple to regularly monitor your pH at home, (or see order form on last page).

The tendency to overacidity is called acidosis which can be caused by such things as kidney, liver or adrenal disorders, improper diet, starvation, anger, stress, fear, fever or excess vitamin C, aspirin or niacin. Symptoms may include insomnia, water retention, migraine headaches, frequent sighing, abnormally low blood pressure, dry hard stools, alternating constipation and diarrhea, sensitivity of the teeth, difficulty swallowing and recessed eyes.

Alkalosis (when the body is too alkaline) can be caused by such things as excessive use of antacids or by poor diet, excessive vomiting (bulimia), endocrine imbalances, high cholesterol, osteo-arthritis, or diarrhea. Symptoms may include drowsiness, protruding eyes, creaking joints, sore muscles, bursitis, edema, night coughs, menstrual problems, allergies, night cramps, chronic indigestion, or asthma.

The first and easiest methods that you can use to correct pH are to increase relaxation, rest, fresh air, and exercise, decrease stress and make dietary adjustments. If you're too acid, decrease acid foods in your diet and eat more alkaline foods; if you're too alkaline, decrease alkaline foods and eat more acid foods. (For a list of acid or alkaline foods see the Appendix at the back of the book).

It's extremely important to monitor your pH levels during urine therapy because if your urine is too alkaline, it may decrease its antibacterial activity. On the other hand, if the urine is consistently exces-

sively acidic, urine therapy could create too much of an acid burden in your body.

In this case, make certain that your diet is primarily alkaline-promoting foods, so that you are balancing your pH and not adding to your body's acid burden through ingesting extremely acidic urine. Also, if you have a severe chronic problem with acidosis **(this is often true of diabetics),** use only a few drops of urine at a time, or substitute a homeopathic urine preparation as described in the section on Homeopathy and Urine in this chapter.

Test your urine pH once or twice each day for a few days when using urine therapy for the first time or when using it intensively. Do not ingest the same urine that you dip the pH strip into for testing. If you are taking only a small maintenance dose per day, test pH once every three to five days in order to determine whether dietary adjustments are needed.

If you find that your urine pH is very acid, add a pinch of baking soda to the urine you'll be ingesting to reduce the acidity.

7. DO NOT USE URINE THERAPY IF YOU ARE PREGNANT WITHOUT A DOCTOR'S SUPERVISION:

Although pregnant women have been treated with successfully urine therapy for morning sickness or edema, the therapy should not be used during pregnancy without the supervision of a doctor familiar with the medical use of urine.

Doctors have reported that they have used urine therapy for morning sickness in pregnancy with excellent results, but there are reports of two spontaneous abortions which occurred after urine therapy treatments (Dunne and Plesch), possibly because of the natural release of toxins which occur with urine therapy.

Fertility: On the other hand, if you're trying to get pregnant, several successful fertility drugs such as Pergonal are made from urine extracts and a few women have reported to me that they feel urine therapy helped them to conceive. The best and safest method in this case is to use urine therapy for a certain time period (six months) before trying to conceive and to discontinue its use during the days that you're attempting to conceive. You can use urine diagnostic tests to determine when you're ovulating and when you've conceived, and you can gear your use of urine accordingly.

Urine Therapy and Drugs: In the past I have recommended that you do not use urine therapy if you are taking any type of drugs or are a heavy smoker, alcohol user or coffee drinker. However, new research has come to my attention that shows that urine therapy can be beneficial under all of these conditions. Dr. William Hitt, an American doctor who actually has urine therapy clinics in Mexico, has reported to me that he has treated 20,000 patients in a 2 1/2 year period with urine therapy injections.

These patients include those with cancer, asthma and other diseases and also patients with severe alcoholism, drug and smoking addictions. Dr. Hitt reports startling success with **no side effects** in using urine injections for addictive disorders and also in combination with prescription drugs. The amount of drugs or contaminants passed into urine is so infinitesimal that they pose no threat and, in fact, appear to act as vaccine-type agents which improve or cure these types of disorders. This is also supported by the book *Urinalysis in Clinical Laboratory Practice* from Miles Laboratories, in which the authors state that even in a case of severe mercury poisoning, the actual amount of mercury passed into the urine is infinitesimal.

When these types of conditions are present, start on 1 - 5 drops orally per day for 3-5 days in order to avoid heavy detoxification. Increase the drops by one or two each day according to how well you're tolerating the therapy, gradually increase the amount as needed to obtain results for your individual condition.

8. IMPROVE YOUR DIET AND AVOID MEAT WHEN USING URINE THERAPY INTENSIVELY AND BEFORE FASTING

In general, your diet should consist of balanced amounts of whole grains, fresh vegetables and small amounts of lean meats and fish. If you are eating large amounts of refined foods, sugar, soda, coffee, etc. you will not get the full benefits of urine therapy and, depending on how poor your diet is, you may experience unpleasant symptoms of headache, nausea, etc., as your body recirculates and expels undesirable elements.

[handwritten margin note: Optimal Diet: Whole grains, fresh vegetables, and small amounts of lean meats & fish. — Especially for intensive therapy]

If you're only using a few oral drops of urine or ingesting one or two ounces once a day, your meat intake can remain normal as long as your usual intake is moderate.

As studies on urea and the kidney have shown (Dr. C. Giordano), urea helps your body break down proteins more efficiently, which may mean that when using urine therapy, you can get the increased benefits

177

of protein intake even though you are eat-ing less meat and other sources of protein.

This information will probably also be of value to vegetarians who rely on much less concentrated protein sources in their foods than regular meat eaters. Decrease or eliminate meat in your diet while ingesting large amounts of urine or preparing for a fast, as combining intensive urine therapy and high meat intake may lead to excess acid levels in the body.

9. DETOXIFYING SYMPTOMS

When you first begin urine therapy, you may initially experience symptoms such as headache, nausea, diarrhea, tiredness, or skin rashes. In many of the research studies in Chapter 4, the doctors often observed such symptoms in their patients, which are the body's natural responses as stored toxins from illness and disorders are excreted and removed from the body.

These symptoms normally disappear within 24 to 36 hours. Also, by starting your therapy with a few oral drops, you may avoid or lessen the severity of detoxification. If you have begun your therapy with larger amounts, and are experiencing unpleasant symptoms, decrease the amount you are ingesting and continue with smaller doses.

Homeopathic remedies and simple herbs can also be used and are often of great help during detoxification to relieve headache, nausea, diarrhea, etc.

10. CHILDREN

Several research studies, such as those done by Drs. Krebs, Plesch, Duncan, Lewis and Dunne, (see Chapter 4), deal specifically with the treatment of children with urine therapy. The easiest internal form of the therapy for children is oral drops of the child's own fresh urine. As mentioned in the studies, for acute flu, colds, viral infections, measles, mumps, chicken pox, etc., small frequent oral doses of 1-10 drops during illness have been shown to be very effective.

For allergies, the research studies indicate that several drops of fresh urine should be given orally before and after meals containing allergenic foods, or when allergic symptoms are present. Drs. Dunne and Lewis give very specific, simple instructions for using urine therapy for treating allergies in children which are included in their reports in Chapter 4.

Another very effective method recommended by Dr. Dunne is to prepare a homeopathic dilution of the child's urine for use throughout the illness or allergy attack. Collect urine at the onset of symptoms and prepare according to the instructions given in the section *Homeopathy and Urine Therapy* further on in this chapter.

Research studies also indicate that symptoms of illness may temporarily increase immediately following the first few doses of urine therapy, but, in all cases, these symptoms dissipated within 24 - 48 hours.

For ear infections, fresh, warm urine drops in the affected ear can give excellent and often instantaneous results. Repeat as needed.

DOSAGE

MAINTENANCE DOSE

A daily maintenance dose is usually considered by those who use urine therapy regularly to be one to two ounces of morning midstream urine. but this dose may also be as little as 5-10 drops per day, or every other day, depending on your individual condition and needs. Many lifetime users of urine therapy such as the former prime minister of India, have commented that regular use of urine therapy noticeably assists in maintaining energy levels, reducing aging and in preventing illness.

SEVERE, ACUTE AND CHRONIC ILLNESSES

For those with chronic or severe illnesses such as cancer, some urine therapy users such as John Armstrong strongly recommend ingesting as much urine as you pass or as much as possible during the day for several days, however, much smaller doses have also been reported to be effective (see Personal Testimonials in Chapter 7).

If you are ingesting large amounts, fasting or sharply decreasing your solid food intake during this time reduces the burden on the kidneys and allows the body to use more energy for healing, rather than digestion.

It would be extremely unadvisable for most people to undertake the kind of prolonged urine fast that John Armstrong suggests, and short

fasting

therapy

"cleansing

urine and water fasts of one to three days can be very effective. Stop ingestion shortly before bed at night so that the body can rest, and resume when you awake in the morning.

If you do not want to fast, but feel that you need to ingest larger amounts of urine, eat small, simple, light meals, preferably, fresh home-made unseasoned vegetable soups.

If you feel you need a grain, use plain millet or rice, or whole grain, salt-free crackers. There is more information on fasting further on in this chapter.

Long-standing, difficult conditions naturally may require a longer peri-od of treatment. What I discovered in my own treatment was that I needed to ingest a large amount initially (about 2 ounces 4-5 times/day) every day, for about two weeks, at which point, I switched to small frequent doses (one to two ounces) three to four times a day for another two weeks and then tapered off to 1-2 ounces twice a day, then every other day, etc. The maintenance dose is 5-10 drops per day. This was my approach, but you may find that your individual require-ments are more or less than these amounts.

If you are suffering from an acute illness such as an infection, the tradi-tional treatment is to fast completely or to eat only light meals such as homemade, unseasoned vegetable broth while ingesting frequent doses of urine for at least one day, or until you feel that your improvement is complete and stable. I have found, as have many others, that eating heavily too soon after recovering from a viral or bacterial infection may produce a relapse, so make sure that you're feeling stable before start-ing to eat normally again.

Always break your fast by slowly reintroducing light foods, homemade fresh vegetable soups, then crackers, grains, etc. (See page 182.)

REST, REST, REST

charlie

Once you have healed a serious illness and achieved improved health, continue the practice of a daily maintenance dose of urine therapy and a good diet. Also, never allow yourself to become consistently exhaust-ed or overtired. Consistent proper rest is much more crucial to health than most people realize. And once you have recovered from a major illness, you must be extremely vigilant in getting abundant rest and relaxation.

I have seen many instances in which people completely cure them-selves of even 'incurable' diseases through urine therapy and natural healing and remain well for a number of years, only to completely undo all the good they've accomplished by over-confidently pushing themselves to extremes in their work or recreation.

Exercise APPROPRIATELY

One of the saddest examples of this error that I know of was the case of a young, bright, determined AIDS patient who had completely cured himself of all visible and clinical evidence of the disease, but subsequently consistently and relentlessly overworked at his demanding corporate job. Eventually, he fell ill, relapsed and was not able to recover. However, in another case, a person who had recovered from a serious illness experienced a relapse from overexertion, but complete rest and intense urine therapy led to an excellent recovery. But why put yourself through that ordeal and risk the chance of seriously undermining your body's hard-won repair work?

(everything) that can be done can be undone, good and bad alike.

Assiduous urine therapy can give you such renewed vigor and energy, that it's easy to become overconfident and overdo, which, is not a huge problem for normal people. But for people recovering from major illnesses, exhaustion can pose a life-long threat, so protect your newfound health and your natural immune defenses with lots of rest, fresh air, moderate exercise and minimized stress.

KIDNEY DISORDERS

If you have a history or presence of a kidney infection, limit the initial amount of oral urine therapy you take to small doses such as 1-5 drops once or twice a day, or use a homeopathic dilution as described in the section on Homeopathy and Urine Therapy in this chapter. Decrease or eliminate meat ingestion and acid-forming foods before beginning the therapy. Also, check your acidity levels with pH strips, and begin urine therapy when your acid levels have normalized or decreased substantially. (Refer to research studies on treatment of nephritis, and kidney disorders, in the Index. See also sections on Acid/Alkaline balancing in the Appendix and the Question and Answer section in this chapter).

ALLERGIES

In the clinical research studies done on urine therapy and allergies, practitioners such as Dunne and Wilson used oral drops with excellent results. Refer to these studies for directions and again, begin with one or two drops and then gradually increase the number of drops, or as Wilson suggests, take the drops until you can no longer sense the urine taste or temperature. If you know what your allergies are, take the drops before eating a food that you're allergic to; if you don't know what you're allergic to, take several drops of fresh urine immediately upon the appearance of symptoms, and repeat this method each time the symptoms re-occur.

Homeopathic urine preparations, as described by Dr. Dunne, are also excellent for allergies, as you can preserve the urine collected at the height of allergy symptoms for long term treatment of the allergy. See the section on preparing homeopathic urine in this chapter.

FOOD POISONING

Several of the research studies show that urea is a proven anti-bacterial agent (Drs. Schlegel, Kaye, Weinstein etc.), and urine has been found to contain antibodies to food contaminants such as salmonella bacteria in infected individuals (Lerner and Remington). Begin by taking 1-5 drops. Increase dosage as tolerated.

FASTING

Fasting on urine is an excellent therapy that can produce extraordinary results, especially for intractable diseases and tough chronic conditions, but always work into a fast slowly. Begin with oral drops for two to three weeks, increase your dosage to 1- 3 ounces during the next two or three weeks, and begin fasting the following week. Eliminate all meat intake at least three days before the fast.

When I first started urine therapy, I was so seriously ill with so many different conditions and in such extreme pain, that I rushed into a week-long fast on urine and water alone. But I don't recommend this approach because I've found that it isn't necessary to rush into the therapy in order to get good results. Pushing your body too quickly can produce often severe detoxifying symptoms such as headaches, fever, nausea, depression, or fatigue that you can lessen or avoid by simply adjusting to the therapy gradually with a few oral drops each day.

During the fast, ingest as much urine as you pass during the day until it becomes completely clear; stop ingesting for a few hours and then resume. Decrease or stop your intake at night and begin again when you awake in the morning.

Alternate urine intake with small sips of cool water or ice-chips if desired. Drink as much water as you feel thirsty for, and stay well-hydrated at all times, but do not force-drink large quantities of water; as research shows (Kaye and Schlegel), this can dilute the urine, and decrease the urea's anti-bacterial action. Force-drinking water, in addition to urine ingestion, may also stress the kidneys.

Combine urine fasting with urine skin massages, particularly on the face, neck and feet. John Armstrong insisted on this method because he felt that it gave extra nourishment to the body while fasting and eliminated possible headaches and nausea. The rubs are also refreshing and make the skin clear and soft.

When breaking the fast, start by eating a simple homemade fresh vegetable soup broth such as one made of fresh kale, carrots, fresh green leeks, scallion tops and a little fresh ginger. Do not add salt or seasonings. Eat only the broth for a day or two, the broth and vegetable the next day, and begin gradually adding in more vegetables and carbohydrates such as rice and millet over the next few days.

Short periods of fasting (1-3 days) can be an extremely effective method for cleansing and healing the body; long fasts should always be undertaken with caution and supervision.

HOMEOPATHY AND URINE THERAPY

In the course of using urine therapy, I found that combining the therapy with homeopathic medicines in particular can produce incredible results, even for the toughest, most stubborn chronic conditions. Severely weakened, debilitated, chronically ill individuals often develop extreme sensitivities to ordinarily helpful herbal, vitamin, mineral and other medicinal preparations, but are able to tolerate homeopathic medicines very well.

Homeopathic medicines are simply extremely diluted natural substances such as plants, minerals, etc. that gently stimulate a healing reaction in the body. A homeopathic medicine is prepared by diluting a minute amount of a particular natural substance with water; the dilution is shaken several times and then alcohol may be added to the solution as a preservative. You can take the homeopathic medicine in its liquid form, or as a small sucrose pill which has been saturated with the liquid.

HOMEOPATHIC URINE

Dr. Nancy Dunne, the allergy researcher, reported that her colleague, Dr. Fife, used urine in the form of a homeopathic dilution with excellent results. Homeopathic urine is excellent for children and may be helpful to those with extreme sensitivities. It also provides a means of preserv-

Dr. Dunne reported that the following procedure for preparing a homeopathic dose of urine was used by Dr. Fife, and had produced remarkable healing:

1. To 5 mls (1/6 of an ounce) of distilled water in a sterile bottle add one drop of fresh urine.

2. Cap the bottle and shake vigorously 50 times (this is the first dilution).

3. Take one drop of this mix and add to another 5 mls (1/6 oz.) of distilled water; shake 50 times.

4. Take one drop of this mix and add to 5 mls (1/6 oz.) of 80 to 90 proof vodka which acts as a preservative.

5. Place three drops under the tongue hourly until there is obvious improvement or temporary exacerbation of symptoms. As improvement progresses, lengthen the interval between treatments. After 3 days, suspend treatment to avoid pushing the immune system. Treatment is resumed if progress remains static or relapse occurs.

ing urine collected during the first stages or the onset of illness, at which time the urinary antibodies and immune defense agents are most reported to be most numerous and active.

Pre-prepared homeopathic urea can also be purchased, although this would contain only urea and none of the antibodies or immune factors of a whole urine homeopathic preparation.

The traditional book for selecting and using homeopathic medicines is referred to as the *Materia Medica*, which contains a listing of the remedies and indications for their use. These lists are referred to as Repertories, such as Boericke's Repertory and Kent's Repertory. These books are actually very enjoyable to learn to use, and the Boericke's Repertory in particular can guide you to very specific, effective remedies for virtually every disorder.

For beginners who feel unsure about how to use homeopathy, the best book I have found as an overall introduction to self-care through homeopathy is *The Family Guide to Homeopathy, Symptoms and Natural Solutions*, by Dr. Andrew Lockie. This is a tremendously comprehensive self-help guide which introduces the fundamentals of how the body functions, how and why specific illnesses and disorders are contracted, and what homeopathic remedies will best augment the body's natural healing. This book is an extraordinary adjunct to urine therapy and contains helpful material about a wide range of disorders that I have never found anywhere else.

When using homeopathy, you have a choice of two different dilutions referred to as "x" potencies or "c" potencies. The "x" potencies are sold commercially in health food stores, etc. I have found that the c potencies are excellent for home use, as their effect seems more pronòunced than the commercial preparations; many homeopathic doctors also prefer the c potencies.

Homeopathic medicines are safe and produce no side effects. These medicines are considered to be FDA approved, because they were widely used in the U.S. earlier in the century and so were "grandfathered" in to the FDA list of approved medical treatments; some homeopathic remedies are sold in health food stores or can be obtained from a homeopathic doctor or catalog.

Combining homeopathy with urine therapy was, for me, incredibly effective for a wide variety of serious disorders as well as for mild disorders such as headaches, colds, indigestion, etc. For more information on using homeopathy with urine therapy, you can also refer to the book I've written on the subject entitled, *Healing Yourself with Homeopathy*.

EXTERNAL USE

SKIN APPLICATIONS

Applying urine to the skin is an excellent treatment for every imaginable type of skin disorder including all rashes, eczema, psoriasis, acne, etc. The urea in urine, as the research studies demonstrated, is also excellent for cosmetic use as an overall skin beautifier and moisturizer.

1. Use either fresh or old urine for skin applications, although old urine has a higher ammonia content and has been found to be more effective in treating many stubborn skin disorders such as eczema or psoriasis.

2. When treating skin disorders such as eczema, psoriasis, rashes, etc. pour a small amount of urine onto a cotton ball or pad and pat or massage it lightly onto the affected area, making sure that the area is well saturated.

3. Discard the pad and saturate another clean pad with fresh urine and reapply, lightly patting and soaking the affected area. Continue reapplying in this manner for 5-10 minutes or as many times as desired – the more that the affected area is treated, the better.

4. Secure a clean soaked pad to the affected area with a gauze or cotton wrap and leave secured for several hours for additional healing. These urine packs are also incredibly effective for any type of insect sting, bite or poison oak or ivy. (See Urine Packs and Compresses).

5. Another method is to pour old or fresh urine into clean, plastic spray bottle and spray the rash, eczema, etc.

SKIN MASSAGES

Always augment your use of oral urine therapy with skin massages particularly on the face, neck and feet. John Armstrong recommended this practice especially when fasting for an acute condition, and people who use it, swear by it. These massages have a tonifying, refreshing, relaxing effect and are said to allow for gradual absorption of urine nutrients through the skin.

Pour either old or fresh urine into a wide, shallow container and dip your hands into the liquid. Shake off excess, then vigorously massage into a small area of skin anywhere on the body until hands and skin are dry. Rewet hands and begin massaging another area until dry; repeat this step until all skin areas have been well massaged. Rinse with warm water.

Do not attempt these massages on extremely elderly or infirm individuals. Also, make certain that you use normal urine for massages. If your own urine is dark, turbid or abnormal looking, wait until you have used the urine internally over the course of two or three days, at which time the urine usually appears clear and can then be used for massages. Urine from a normal healthy person other than yourself may also be used for your external massage.

If you are a heavy smoker, or are taking therapeutic or recreational drugs, do not use your own urine externally or internally (or use only **extremely small** amounts).

COSMETIC APPLICATIONS

1. For cosmetic use or moisturizing, pour a very small amount of normal fresh urine or urine which has been stored for a day or two into your hand and massage lightly into the skin until dry; then pour additional urine into your hand, massage it into another area of the skin until dry and so on.

2. Rinse well with warm water when completed, but wash without soap. Your skin is naturally slightly acidic, and this natural acidity is usually destroyed by soaps which are all alkaline and diminish the skin's natural protective acid mantle.

3. You can apply a moisturizer after the massage, but make sure that it's a simple, natural one that doesn't contain lot of drying alcohol or other chemicals. Also, you can add a few drops of urine to a small amount of your moisturizing cream each time you apply the cream.

As the research studies show, urea replenishes the water content of the skin because it binds hydrogen and attracts moisture to the skin in a way that no mineral oil or glycerin-based lotions or creams can.

You'll be absolutely amazed at the softness and beauty of your skin after even one treatment with a urine massage. Old dead skin immediately flakes away, and your skin becomes wonderfully soft, rosy and with time, even wrinkles will disappear. Urine massages have also been reported to eliminate varicose veins and cysts on the skin (see Personal Testimonials).

URINE PACKS AND COMPRESSES

SKIN DISORDERS

Urine packs give added healing to skin disorders such as eczema, psoriasis, athlete's foot, ringworm, poison ivy and oak, etc. in addition to urine massages and soaks:

1. Soak gauze bandages or cotton balls in fresh or old urine and place them over the affected areas.

2. Cover the urine pack with light plastic (like Saran-wrap) and tie in place with gauze strips.

3. Try to keep the pack on as long as possible, especially with more severe conditions. Add additional urine to the pack with a medicine dropper every few hours to keep the pack wet.

BITES AND STINGS

Urine packs are tremendously useful and effective for relieving the discomfort of all insect bites and stings.

When I first moved to Arizona, I was stung on the foot by a scorpion. My foot immediately swelled to almost double its size and was unbelievably painful. I dragged myself into the house, applied a soaked urine pack and tied it in place. Within 15 minutes, the pain had disappeared and the swelling had lessened considerably. I kept the pack on overnight, and when I removed it in the morning, the swelling and redness had completely disappeared. The pain and irritation of bee stings and mosquito bites is also wonderfully relieved by this method.

SNAKE BITE

Urine packs should also be used immediately for poisonous snake bites. Follow emergency first-aid instructions to incise the wound and remove venom if possible. Then apply fresh normal urine to the wound and secure a well-soaked urine pack over it. Keep pack wet until medical help can be obtained.

GROWTHS AND TUMORS

Armstrong reported in great length on the remarkable effects of urine compresses in reducing and eradicating a wide variety of internal and external tumors, cysts and abnormal growths.
1. Compresses should be used in combination with internal urine therapy for treating any type of abnormal growth.

2. In preparing a compress, use a thick pad of clean white folded cotton material (such as an old T-shirt).

3. Soak the pad in a container of fresh or old urine. Warm the urine by pouring it into a glass container, then place the jar in a container of hot water. While lying down, place wet compress over the affected area and cover with a clean folded towel. Keep the compress applied for as long as possible, reapplying warm urine as needed to keep the compress wet. Urine compresses have also been reported to be effective for many internal disturbances and for arthritic and rheumatic pains.

WOUNDS, BURNS AND ABRASIONS

As so many research and clinical studies have shown, urea is a tremendously effective anti-bacterial agent and an excellent healing treatment for wounds and burns of all types. Use fresh, normal urine for treating open wounds.

1. Saturate a thick gauze bandage or cotton pad with fresh urine, place it over the wound or burn and secure it with additional gauze; cover with plastic or soft towel to prevent leakage.

2. Reapply fresh urine with clean medicine dropper directly onto the existing inside compress. Reapply fresh compress as often as possible. Urine is also known to prevent scarring, so keep the urine pack applied as long or as often as possible until healing is complete.

Many people have applied urine compresses to burns and cuts with amazing results. The pain is quickly relieved and the burn or wound heals rapidly without scarring.

EYE AND NOSE DROPS

There are reports from people who have used urine drops for both eye and nose drops, for relief of eye itching or inflammation, or for nasal congestion. In both cases, make certain that you are using fresh, clear, normal urine only and that the acidity factor of the urine is normal (see previous section on Monitoring Your pH in this chapter). Also, make certain that the eye dropper you use for the eye drops is sterilized. A compress of fresh normal urine is also excellent for external eye inflammations such as styes.

QUESTIONS AND ANSWERS ABOUT URINE THERAPY

1. CAN MY DOCTOR ADMINISTER UREA, AS THE RESEARCHERS IN THE STUDIES DID?

The urine extract, urea, is FDA approved and can be administered by your doctor. A Physician's Guide to Your Own Perfect Medicine is available if your doctors would like additional information contained in the research studies on the clinical application of urea. As the research studies indicate, oral or injected urea has been shown to be extremely effective and safe in treating cases where excess fluid production is a problem (see pgs. 99-103). Urea's anti-bacterial, anti-viral and diuretic properties are also well established by the research findings in Chapter 4.

Using urea in conjunction with natural urine therapy can be discussed with your doctor, once he or she has been made aware of the research findings relating to urea and urine therapy.

2. WHAT ABOUT URINE INJECTIONS?

Many people have asked me about the efficacy of urine injections, and as you've seen, many of the research studies presented in Chapter 4 utilized injections of urine as part of the therapy. But doctors have also used oral urine or urea therapy in non-emergency cases with equally good results and urine injections have the reported side effect of occasional redness and swelling at the site of the injection which doesn't occur, of course, with oral therapy.

Oral urine therapy also allows for slower application and absorption which can decrease any possible de-toxifying symptoms. Injections deliver an abrupt, forced introduction of medicinal substances into the body, without allowing for the body's gradual adjustment to the substance. However, there really isn't any need for this sudden forcing of a medicinal substance into the body unless there is an emergency situation that requires it.

Gradual introduction of urine therapy, or any medical therapy is always important, but even more so if you have a history of poor nutrition or chronic, serious illnesses which weaken the body and promote poisons and toxins in the system. Introducing a new therapy too rapidly places a strain on an already weakened system and can cause a sudden release of toxins that may make you feel ill unnecessarily.

As clinical studies have demonstrated, oral urine or urea can be just as effective for non-emergency cases as injected urine. And, as doctors themselves have commented, oral urine therapy can be used at safely and effectively at home without the unnecessary cost and inconvenience of a doctor's office visit, while injections can be reserved for those with urgent needs under a doctor's care.

However, if your situation is extremely severe, urine injections can definitely be of benefit. Dr. William Hitt (whom I mentioned earlier) runs two urine therapy clinics in Mexico and has administered hundreds of thousands of injections to severely ill patients with remarkable success. For more information on Dr. Hitt's clinics call 1-800-800-8849.

4. CAN TOO MUCH URIC ACID OR UREA BE HARMFUL?

As several of the clinical studies showed, urea, even in large doses, has been found to be harmless to the body.

Researchers, (Urea – New Use of An Old Agent), reported that they safely administered urea daily to several patients for a period ranging from several days to weeks, and in some cases, even several months, without any side effects, in doses ranging from 100 mg. per kilogram of body weight to as much as 600 mg. per kilogram of body weight. Decaux, et. al, (5-Year Treatment of SIADH with Oral Urea), prescribed 30 grams/day for more than 5 years for a patient with excess water and salt retention (hyponatremia), and occasionally prescribed doses up to 60-90 grams per day for one or two days without side effects.

Normal urine contains approximately 2% urea, and you normally excrete about 24.5 grams/day, which is well below the dosages just mentioned. So even if you ingested all of the urine you passed during the day, (approximately 25 grams of urea), this amount is much less than the dosages mentioned above, especially in view of the fact that you would not be ingesting all the urine you pass every day for long periods of time.

Uric acid, usually thought to be a toxic waste product of the body, has been found by researchers to actually be a natural body defense against cancer and aging, allowing us to live much longer than other mammals (Omni Magazine article, 1982). Most people think that uric acid causes gout, but strictly speaking, it is not the uric acid alone that causes the gout, but rather an overall, ongoing and chronic overacidity in the body which can be caused by many different factors including improper, overly-acid diet, kidney, liver and adrenal disorders, obesity, diabetes, chronic stress, undereating (anorexia), etc.

Normally, the amount of uric acid contained in urine is not a problem during urine therapy, because the body will excrete the amount it does not need. However, when the body's ability to excrete excess acids is impaired, uric acid excretion is, of course, also impaired.

If you feel that you have a problem with chronic, ongoing overacidity (see section on Monitoring Acid/Alkaline Levels in this chapter), **make certain that you decrease or eliminate meat while using urine therapy. Also, improve your diet by eating more alkaline foods, and decreasing acid foods before and after you start on urine therapy.** Monitor your acid/alkaline level with pH strips to determine when your pH has returned to a normal or more balanced condition.

In cases of chronic acidosis (over-acidity), do not do extended urine fasts or ingest large quantities over long periods of time. Use oral drops to begin; start with 1-2 drops once a day,and gradually increase to 5-10 drops two to four times a day, for one to three weeks, depending on your need. Monitor your pH levels and your symptoms (see symptoms of acidosis in this chapter). You can also dilute the urine in water, or use a homeopathic preparation of your urine (see section on Homeopathy and Urine Therapy in this chapter).

5. HOW LONG SHOULD I USE URINE THERAPY?

The amount of time needed to achieve results with urine therapy is different for every person and each condition. Many people have found that chronic, long-standing complaints require a longer period of time to heal, while others experience rapid results. Logically speaking, it probably depends on the condition of your body's immune functions, ability to repair itself, amount of damage to the body that has been sustained during illness, etc.

In general, do not use large amounts of urine internally for more than two to three weeks at a time. Once you have achieved solid results at whatever dose you're taking, begin decreasing the amount and number of days that you use the therapy internally, and use only a maintenance dose from then on, unless you come down with a cold, infection, etc., at which time you would increase your dosage amount and frequency during the period of illness.

A maintenance dose for many people is one to two ounces of morning urine per day, although **even 2-5 drops of morning urine per day or every other day could be considered a good maintenance dose, especially for those with acidosis or weak kidneys.**

6. CAN I DO DIAGNOSTIC URINE TESTS AT HOME?

There are several excellent urine testing kits that have been developed in the last few years that can be used at home and can save you an amazing amount of time and money.

Now you can perform many of the same urine tests at home that your doctor performs in his office. Also, these tests are particularly helpful when using urine therapy because you can monitor your own health progress easily and inexpensively.

Urine home test strips are available to test for these conditions and many others:

- Kidney and Urinary Tract Infections
- Diabetes
- Blood in the urine
- Pregnancy
- Ovulation
- Liver Function

You can purchase these strips in drugstores or they are available by catalog.

The booklet, *Simple Diagnostic Tests You Can Do at Home* gives a wide range of information on what tests are available, how to use them, and how to interpret these tests.

The booklet also explains how to interpret your urine color and appearance which are important additional indicators of health conditions.

8. CAN PETS BE TREATED WITH URINE THERAPY?

Many of the research tests on urine recycling have been undertaken with animals, and veterinarians have used urine therapy for treatment by catherizing the animal and administering oral urine drops with reportedly good results.

SUMMARY

Remember to **begin your treatment slowly with a few oral drops** and increase the amount to a well-tolerated dosage.

Make sure that you're eating well and decreasing your meat intake as you increase your urine intake. Do not use the therapy while ingesting heavy amounts of nicotine, caffeine or while using recreational drugs or therapeutic drugs than small amounts. If you do decide to use it, however, use only very small amounts (3-5 drops 1x day.)

Frequent small doses of one to three ounces for two to three weeks can be extremely effective; larger amounts can be taken for several days if needed and if you have no history or presence of kidney disease; gradually decrease the amount once your symptoms have abated and healing is apparent.

Drink as much water as you feel thirsty for, and keep well-hydrated, but do not force-drink large amounts of fluid during the therapy. Do not fast for long periods of time without competent, professional supervision.

Daily maintenance doses vary from a few drops to one to two ounces of morning urine, depending on your sensitivity and preference.

THE DO'S AND DON'TS OF URINE THERAPY (UT)

DO:

1. Start with small amounts and work up to larger amounts gradually for internal use.

2. Use only fresh urine internally.

3. Test your pH to make certain that you are not overly acidic before using the therapy and continue to monitor your pH periodically during internal use of UT.

DO NOT:

1. Rush into the therapy with large amounts.

2. DO NOT combine urine therapy with a starvation diet (or fasting) unless you have been using the therapy for at least two months.

3. DO NOT continue to work while fasting on UT. If you are ingesting large amounts of UT and fasting, you must rest and relax in order to avoid possibly stressing the kidneys.

4. DO NOT ingest large amounts while eating a consistently acidic diet.

CHAPTER 7

SPECIFIC DISORDERS

There are many excellent testimonials and case studies on specific illnesses that have already been mentioned throughout the book, which you can refer to by looking in the Index under the name of the specific disorder that concerns you.

I'll also mention a few more personal stories here as they relate to specific illnesses. These stories are taken from personal letters that I have read or from other published collections of testimonials on urine therapy, in particular, The Miracles of Urine Therapy, by Margie Adelman and Beatrice Barnett, and an Indian publication, Practical Guide to Auto Urine Therapy, by Acharya Jagdish. The stories are listed under specific condition titles, but many of the individual stories report on a number of different conditions, so you might want to read through all of them if your particular disorder does not appear to be mentioned.

Also, if you'd like to read more personal testimonials, I highly recommend John Armstrong's book, The Water of Life which is replete with inspiring stories of remarkable cures with urine therapy, although his method of strict, long-term fasting of one to two months is extremely radical, and should never be undertaken without supervision.

Your specific condition may not be mentioned here, but that doesn't mean that urine therapy can't help you. Urine contains such a huge array of medicinally valuable elements, many of which have not even as yet been identified, that its use is indicated in all approaches to healing.

Even if feel that you're in good health, a small maintenance dose of urine therapy provides excellent energy-promoting nutrients, hormones, enzymes, etc., as well as purported longevity agents such as DHEA that everyone can benefit from, while natural urine antibodies enhance preventive health care and contribute to overall and lasting good health.

Personal Testimonials

AIDS

Mr. B. – Age 38. HIV positive. T4 210. Lympodenopathy, mild fatigue, severe acne on back. Commenced urine therapy and gland swelling reduced entirely within 48 hours of treatment. Fatigue gone within days. Acne dissipated dramatically over the following two weeks and more so once topical application of urine was begun – three week course of tetracycline (500 mg. 4 x/day) had negligible results. When urine therapy is skipped for more than two days, gland swelling and fatigue return. After urine therapy, I am feeling much better, normal again. No other treatment used. I am so grateful for this gift of life.

Mr. M. – 46 years old. T4 160. Heavy night sweats and fatigue (18 hours of sleep a day) for three months prior to urine therapy. Symptoms totally resolved within 10 days. Skin had taken on a dry, ashy look which was also resolved. Within 2 weeks of treatment, was playing one-hour games of basketball daily. No other treatment used (or available) for treating symptoms.

Mr. R.B. – 32 years of age. T4 210. T4/T8 ratio .3. Commenced urine therapy and mild fatigue and dizziness dissipated over a month. At 32 oz./day, experienced some diarrhea and cramps. Cut back to 8 oz. every 8 hrs. Lymph gland swelling has reduced by more than 50%. For over a year before urine therapy, experienced intense eye itching. A few drops of fresh urine in the eyes stops the itching immediately. Regular use of urine therapy prevents return of fatigue.

Mr. L. – I am a PWA (person with Aids). My only symptom was a low T-cell count. I have been doing urine-therapy for four months now. My last test showed that my t-cell count went up from 285 to 489.

Mr. M. – I am a PWA. My major problem was parasites. My stool sample contained pus, large amounts of yeast and several parasites. After urine therapy, my last test came back totally clear. No more pus and no more parasites.

As discussed earlier in the book, the medically proven anti-viral properties of urea could possibly be enhanced through administration of urea extract (which is an FDA approved treatment) in addition to natural urine therapy. Consult with your doctor on using urea orally or by injection, to augment urine therapy in treating AIDS.

The anti-viral, anti-bacterial and diuretic properties of urea have been repeatedly proven and could certainly be of tremendous value in treating the HIV virus and the concomitant bacterial and viral infections, excess fluid production, etc. As the clinical studies conducted by the researchers in the report, Urea – New Use Of An Old Agent, (see research studies) clearly demonstrated, urea, even in extremely large doses, is completely safe, so using it to enhance the activity of natural urine might well produce outstanding results.

CANCER

Dr. V.P. – I am a qualified medical doctor and was diagnosed with cancer of the epiglottis (throat) with enlarged cervical lymph nodes. After receiving chemotherapy and a course of cobalt therapy I was to receive surgery. However, before continuing with conventional treatments, I began using urine therapy. After using urine therapy for more than a month my symptoms disappeared and the proposed surgery was cancelled. I am now leading a fully active professional life.

Mr. R.R. – I was officially diagnosed with Adenocarcinoma of the chest with possible infiltration of the left lung two years ago. While I was in the hospital because of the concurrent symptoms (collapsed lung with 8 liters of bloody fluid) I was in a desperate struggle to stop production of the fluid.

My bowels had stopped for a period of 5 days. I then came across information on urine therapy. As soon as I ingested my urine it was miraculous. I had five major bowel movements. The relief was incredible and the fluid production subsequently died down, to the doctors amazement. They had no recourse but to remove my chest tube. They wanted to continue with proposed treatments (chemo, radiation, surgery), but I signed out of the hospital.

Needless to say I am still here after two years even though my parents were informed that I had only four months to survive. I employed a number of holistic approaches (colonics, herbs, etc.), but to be perfectly honest I know it was the internal and external use of this therapy that has saved my life. I hope you can circulate my story to others to spread hope through this miracle cure.

Mrs. E. – In the summer of 1983 I was diagnosed with cancer in my spine. I had radiation treatments and the pain subsided. After that I treated myself by natural means. Three years later I became sick again and was diagnosed with metastatic cancer of the liver. My doctors gave me pain killers and told me there was nothing they could do and sent me home. I tried another therapy but in November my condition worsened and I developed hepatitis with high fever and intense pain. I then tried urine therapy. I drank only my first morning urine. By the fifth day I felt more energetic. By the 10th day I returned to the doctor. He could not believe I was still alive. I drink my urine every morning. As of June, my liver is slightly swollen, but I do not have any pain.

This woman's experience is interesting in terms of determining how much urine to ingest in treating cancer. She reports she drank only her morning urine with good results, but the liver swelling later returned, whereas, another woman who reported that she had an inoperable uterine tumor drank all the urine she passed daily for seven days, at which time she reported that the tumor had disappeared, which may be an indication that larger amounts are required for dealing with such disorders.

Mr. L. – Diagnosed with Kaposi's Sarcoma, (form of cancer that often accompanies AIDS), cellulitis and edema. Used urine therapy daily for 3 months internally and externally. He reported that he did not experience any detoxifying symptoms with urine therapy and attributes this to several weeks of high enemas (one a week) taken before beginning urine therapy. He noted that the water retention in his legs disappeared with urine therapy and the major lesions on his legs opened and healed. He found that maintaining a healthy diet and the use of urine (fasting and external applications) has kept his cancer in a prolonged state of remission.

Since 1984 we have been using urine therapy in our practice and have found it beneficial for many diseases ranging from skin problems and even carcinomas. We would welcome more information on urine therapy and would be pleased to participate in an international conference.
Bodylife School of Practical Healing
Netherlands

BURNS

Mrs. B. – One day I wanted to make sure my iron was turned off before I left the house, so I checked the iron surface with the palm of my hand expecting it to be cold. To my surprise, the iron was hot and I burned my hand severely. Then I remembered that some weeks earlier I had stored a bottle containing urine. I used the urine from the bottle and covered my burns with it. The pain soon subsided and a few hours later, my hand looked and felt as though nothing had happened to it. No blisters, no scars and no redness remained.

CANDIDA

Ms. L.M. – My experience with urine therapy was that I was able to solve a difficult chronic yeast infection, as well a chronic constipation problem. Also, I began my menstrual flow after a three year cessation after using urine therapy.

Ms. M.G. – I have had a chronic case of severe candida for many years as a result of taking large doses of antibiotics for a long period for a sinus infection. I tried every drug my doctor would give me, such as Nizoral and Nystatin, and also many herbs, but the candida would not go away and even showed up in blood tests.

Finally, I heard about urine therapy and began drinking it three times a day. After only a few days, the relief was tremendous. The vaginal burning and itching stopped completely, the water weight disappeared, and my energy returned. I've been taking it for some time now, my headaches and general itching are gone, and I feel better than I have in years.

CHILDREN'S COMPLAINTS

Ms. M.D. - I am raising a grandchild who got a very back start in life, she was bombarded with antibiotics for inner ear infections and other problems. With good diet and care she got much better, but she was wide open for eery allergy imaginable, (she had severe skin rashes, scaling, etc.). When she was 2,3, and 4-years-old, she could hardly breathe at night and was always stuffed up.

I started her on three then five drops of her own urine one time per day about a week ago. Let me tell you that this child is a different person. Her nose is completely free of mucus and I can't believe the personality change. From a whiny, clingy irritating child, she is acting happy, attacks her school work with a vigor I never saw before. She sleeps clear through the night, with no restlessness.

CYSTS

Mrs. D. – Was seeking relief from sebaceous cysts which were all over the face and neck. She had the cysts for over a year and had been to many doctors, taken medication and tried countless skin creams. Then she decided to try urine therapy. After rubbing urine on the cysts for about a week, the cysts opened and drained, and new skin began to form. Over a period of three weeks, her skin completely healed. She commented that she now applies urine to her face daily and that her complexion has never looked as good.

COLITIS

Mr. M. – I have been hospitalized three time in the past year for gastrointestinal problems created by my strong negative reactions to antibiotics administered for lung infections. I refused to continue with the medication, however, my rectal bleeding from colitis and internal hemorrhoids continued.

In the meantime, a friend told me that he was familiar, from childhood, with the use of urine enemas for problems such as mine, so I began using urine for daily enemas for a week. By the end of the week, the bleeding had stopped completely and now, several months later, I have not passed a single drop of blood.

DEPRESSION, IMMUNE DEFICIENCY

Mr. D. – I was suffering from an undefined immune deficiency problem. I had many skin problems (rashes and ulcers) and for weeks was running a low grade fever. I always felt tired and very depressed. I could not work and this just added to my problem of financial difficulties from all the doctor bills and medication I had tried.

One night I was extremely depressed. I had heard about urine therapy and, even though I was very skeptical, I tried it. Within a week my energy came back by at least 60%. My diet had not been very good, and after beginning urine therapy, I experienced detoxifying symptoms of rashes and high fever for several days. I realized that my body had been trying to get rid of these toxins through my skin for a long time (which was why I had chronic skin problems), but I had suppressed it with many medications. I continued with the therapy. Today, I am back at work again, the depression is gone and I am a different person.

DIABETES

Miss D. – Reported to have juvenile diabetes. After ingesting urine for about a month, she found that she can eliminate her evening dose of insulin. She tested her blood sugar constantly. About a month later, she reported that she was ready to further reduce her insulin intake. While using urine externally, she also noticed her varicose veins starting to diminish. She is feeling well and has had no other problems while on urine therapy.

Mrs. Kunjama, Bangalore, India – This lady was suffering from diabetes, was overweight and had occasional breathing troubles for about 12 years and had to be frequently hospitalized whenever her temperature ran high every two or three months. Ayurvedic, homeopathic and other medicines had no effect. Insulin injections reduced her suffering to a certain extent, but there was no diminution in her + 2.75 of sugar in her urine at any time.

Mrs. Kunjama began the intake of her own urine as many times as she passed and sipped water. The nurse did the required massage of the body with old urine and helped the lady to wash herself with lukewarm water. On the first day she suffered slightly from diarrhea. After three weeks, her weight was reduced and her breathing trouble ceased. The family doctor was surprised when he detected no trace of sugar in her urine at the end of the treatment.

HEPATITIS B

Mr. R.W. and Mr. R.T. - We are both practitioners of the Natural Health Theory here in Switzerland. Due to the kindness of a close acquaintance of ours in the U.S. we recently received a copy of your most interesting book, Your Own Perfect Medicine, which greatly impressed us. The 'natural medicines theory' with urine is not new to us ... for quite some time now we have been applying this theory as well as doing experimental research work on the subject with extremely positive and successful results. Among other things, for the cure of Hepatitis B, to mention just one point.

LUNG CONDITIONS

Mr. N. – Complained of chest, lung and sinus congestion. After approximately two weeks of both internal and external urine therapy, the congestion disappeared and he was able to breathe easily.

MULTIPLE DISORDERS

Ms. A.R.– I have always tried to take good care of myself, but somehow over the years, several diseases crept up on me. In my 40s and 50s, I developed alopecia areata (extensive hair loss). Later, I developed Rheumatoid Arthritis and Sclerosis (hardening of body and nerve tissues). I also contracted systemic scleroderma (an autoimmune disorder in which the body attacks it own tissues) and Raynaud's Disease (a circulatory disorder that cuts off blood flow to fingers and toes). Epstein-Barr developed, too.

*When the Alopecia began, I would get 3-4 bald spots on my head. My doctor would inject them with cortisone, but eventually I went totally bald. Then I lost all my eyelashes, the hair in my nose and on my arms and legs. It was absolutely horrible . With the Raynaud's, my fingers stung as though they were stuck to ice. I would cry and run hot water over them, but it just came back. I was terribly depressed and really didn't want to live anymore. Then I found out about Your Own Perfect Medicine and decided that I had to try it. I started with one drop a day and then gradually increased to six drops a day after a week. Then I noticed that my fingers were not hurting nearly as much as usual. I started urine therapy in November, 1994. By Feb 1995, I was taking eight large eye droppers and by now I began to see short patches of hair appearing. I continued on the therapy and my hair continued to grow in steadily. On May 29, 1995, off came my wig and I also noticed my eyelashes growing back. By July 1995 I had **all** my hair, eyelashes, nose hair, arms and legs. by September 1995, I was taking 20 large eyedroppers a day, and I now have a beautiful head of hair — thicker than ever. My skin is softer and I feel really good. The Raynaud's symptoms, chronic fatigue, arthritis are all gone. On August 24, 1995, I had a physical — everything was OK! Urine therapy **is** the answer. I thank God every day for this miracle. I want to yell it out to the world!*

MULTIPLE SCLEROSIS

Mr. B.W. – I am extremely thankful for this safe and free method to rid ourselves of many chronic diseases. After using urine therapy, I have improved greatly. My diagnosis of chronic progressive multiple sclerosis has now become something to be cleared away, and not an impenetrable wall as it was before my discovery of urine therapy.

PROSTATE PROBLEMS

Mr. J.S. – I had begun to experience pain and difficulty in urinating in my early thirties, but as I got closer to forty, the problem became much worse and my doctor gave me antibiotics and pain medication, which not only did not improve the situation but actually made the symptoms worse. The doctor told me that he felt that the symptoms were due to a problem with my prostrate. I was going to undergo a battery of tests when a friend told me about auto-urine therapy. I began ingesting just a few drops a couple of times a day, and noticed a decrease in pain on urinating almost immediately. I continued taking small amounts, and then later fasted for about three days. After the fast, all symptoms disappeared. It's been more than a year now, and I am completely free of any pain or problems.

RADIATION THERAPY

Ms. S.G. – I've used UT on my hair for years — in fact all through radiation therapy (aimed just above the eyebrow on the right), I kept my hair. It was a nightly ritual to pour that into my hair (collected in the A.M.), rub cod liver oil into it, wrap with a towel and soak in a hot tub of water!! It works!

RAYNAUD'S SYNDROME

Ms. E.P.– At 78 years old, I have a great abundance of miseries. Recently I developed symptoms of Raynaud's disease and know that the prognosis is grave at best.

I have been on UT about one week following the instructions in your book. My pleasant surprise is that in that short time my symptoms have been reduced 50%.

SURVIVAL, MALARIA

Colonel M.L. – This man first discovered the life-enhancing qualities, as he called them, of urine while serving with the British Army in the western Sahara during World War II. He had become separated from his unit after a night skirmish and had been slightly wounded on the temple by a ricocheting bullet.

When he awoke the following morning, he found himself alone, at the foot of a sand dune with caked blood all over one side of his face and head and his water bottle nearly empty. His first thoughts were of the horrors of dying of thirst. He then recalled that he had been taught in basic training that drinking urine could save one's life in a waterless emergency, and he tried it, saving the last of his water for drinking afterwards.

He drank two-thirds of a cup of urine and used the remainder to moisten his handkerchief which he used as a poultice for his head. He reported that when his platoon members returned to look for him, they had expected to find a corpse and instead found a somewhat parched but cheerful and feverless fighting man who returned to action with his platoon three days later.

When, later in the war, his regiment was sent to the Far East to fight, he contracted malaria which he cured himself in just three days on a urine and water fast, and he reported that he never had a recurrence. He continued to drink his urine every day since that episode, and after nearly 35 years (at age 59) he reported that he was lean, strong and healthy.

VENEREAL DISEASE, PARASITES

Mr. S. – One and one-half months ago I was diagnosed with gonorrhea and herpes. I took medication and the condition improved. But two weeks later the herpes came back and was even worse. I then started urine therapy. Within two or three days, everything cleared up totally. What was even more amazing to me is the parasite problem which I suffered with for quite some time, was inadvertently resolved while treating my herpes.

WEIGHT LOSS

Ms. B. – I not only weighed 198 pounds, but I also had several other health problems including rheumatoid arthritis, severe chronic migraines and an external fungal infection on my foot. I had tried everything to correct these conditions, but nothing had worked.

I heard about urine therapy and tried it externally on my foot, because I had tried every possible medication on the fungal infection with no results. I soaked my foot in urine about three times a day. Five days later, the fungus was gone. My husband thought it was a miracle. Both of us started drinking our urine the very next day and to my surprise, my weight loss speeded up incredibly.

Four and one half months later, I weighed 130 pounds. I lost a total of 68 pounds! My arthritis is gone, my headaches are gone and I feel like I'm 20 years old!

WHOOPING COUGH

Mr. J.R. - When I was 5 or 6 years old I had a whooping cough. The doctor told my mother to give me urine. Two to three days later, my cough was cured and at the same time worms cam out of my body.

WOUNDS

Mr. K. – I was involved in an accident in which a huge rock fell from a height of about four feet directly onto my left foot. I was not wearing closed shoes and the stone ripped almost all the flesh and my toe nail from, luckily, only the middle toe.

As I was traveling in a foreign country, I was unable to get proper medical care and I was extremely worried about infection. I applied an antiseptic creme that I had, but with no results.

After a few days, my toe was an indefinable mass of black and red tissue. Then I met a woman who told me to wrap my foot in a cloth soaked in urine. I did it and was amazed to see how quickly my toe started to heal. New pink skin appeared, pieces of old and damaged skin fell off and within a couple of days, the toe looked nearly normal again. I kept the cloth wet all the time with fresh urine and occasionally with old urine which I collected in a bottle.

Now I have become accustomed to drinking my urine and have my share of the "water of life" every morning.

As I mentioned before, John Armstrong's book, the Water of Life, and Margie Adelman's, Miracles of Urine Therapy, contain many more inspiring testimonials which make extremely interesting and enjoyable reading.

I wish each one of you the very best of health and hope that you, as so many others have done, find renewed health, vigor and long life with your body's own perfect medicine.

Martha Christy

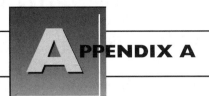

ALKALINE AND ACID FOOD LIST

Alkaline Forming Foods

FRESH VEGETABLES

Artichokes, Asparagus, Avocados, Bamboo Shoots, Beans (String), Beans (wax), Beans, Lima (Dried, or fresh), Beets, Bread, Soy Bean, Cabbage (Red), Carrots, Celery, Chard, Chives, Corn, Cucumbers, Endive, Garlic, Herbs (All), Horse-Radish, Kale, Kohlrabi, Leeks, Lettuce (Leaf), Okra, Onions (Some), Oyster Plant, Parsley, Parsnips, Peas (Fresh), Peppers (Sweet), Pimento, Potatoes (Red), Potatoes (Sweet), Pumpkin, Rutabagas, Sauerkraut, Soy Bean, Spinach (Raw), Sprouts (All), Squash (All kinds, summer), Tomatoes (Yellow), Vegetable Oyster, Watercress, Yams

FRESH FRUITS

Apples (Golden Delicious), Apricots, Berries (All dark), Cherries (Bing), Grapefruit (Pink), Grapes (Flame & Concord, Kumquats, Lemons (Tree Ripened), Mango, Kiwi, Logan Berries, Loquats, Lemon (Ripe), Melons (All kinds), Papaya, Passion Fruit, Peaches (One variety), Pears (Bosc-Japanese)

Acid Forming Foods

FRESH VEGETABLES

Brussel Sprouts, Broccoli, Cauliflower, cabbage, E99 Plant, Lettuce (Iceberg), Mushroom, Potatoes (Red), Radishes, Spinach (Cooked), Tomatoes, Turnips

FRESH FRUITS

Apple (Red & Green), Bananas, Blueberries, Cherries (Light), Coconut, Currants, Cranberries, Dates, Figs, Grapefruit (White), Grapes (Thompson), Limes, Lemons (Picked Green), Nectarines, Olives, Oranges, Peaches (Most), Pears (Bartlett), Persimmons, Pineapple, Plums, Prunes, Pomegranate, Prunes, Raisins, Raspberries, Rhubarb, Quince, Strawberries, Tangerines

Alkaline Forming Foods	Acid Forming Foods
NUTS (RAW)	**NUTS (RAW)**
Cashew, Macadmaia, Pecan	Almonds, Hickory, Pine, Pistachio, Walnuts (Black and English)
STARCHES AND SUGARS	**STARCHES AND SUGARS**
Beans (Pinto), Carob, Corn Bread (Yellow), Corn Meal (Yellow), Corn Meal Cereal, Cornstarch Crackers (Alkaline/whole-grains), Hominy, Soybeans (bread/dried, Spaghetti (Egg Noodle), Popcorn (yellow) Maple Syrup (100% Pure), Pancake (Alkaline Flour), Pastries (Alkaline Flour), Peas (Dried Green), Rice-Brown - organic, Shortgrain, Vegetable Pasta	Banana Squash, Barley, Bran, Bread (Graham), Bread (Rye), Bread (\White), Bread (Whole Wheat), Cereals (All kinds, packaged), cornmeal (White), Crackers (White), Doughnuts, Dressings, Dry Beans (Most), Dry Peas (Yellow), Dumplings (White), Flour (List), Gravies (most kinds), Honey, Hubbard Squash, Jelly (All kinds), Jerusalem Artichokes, Molasses, Pancakes (White), Pastries (White), Peanuts, Peas (Dried white), Potatoes (Brown skin), Preserves (White sugar), Puddings, Pumpkin, Rice (White/Wild/Long grain?Brown), Rye, Soups (Thick), Spaghetti (White), Sugar (All kinds), Syrups (White sugar), Tapioca, Waffles (White), Wheat
FLOURS	**FLOURS**
Artichoke, Chick Pea, Duram Flour, Masa Harina, Millet, Oat, Rye, Semolina, Soy	Brown Rice, Buckwheat, Barley, Gluten Potato, Wholewheat
PROTEINS	**PROTEINS**
Avocados (Ripe), Beans (Pinto), Buttermilk, Catfish (Farm), clams, Cheese (White), Cornish Hen, Duck, Fish (White), Goat Milk (Raw), Lamb, Nuts, Rabbit, Raw Milk, Seeds (Sprouted all), Turtle, Yogurt Plain	Avocados (Hard), Cashews, Catfish, Cheese (Yellow), Cottage Cheese, Crabs, Buck (Wild), Eggs, Fish (Pink), Hazel Nuts, Hickory Nuts, Lentils, Lobster, Meats (Beef/Pork/Veal), Mutton, Olives (Green), Oysters Peanut (Legume), Peanut Butter, Pine Nuts, Pistachio Nuts, Poultry (Chicken), Turkey (Dark meat), Shrimp, Scallops, Squab, Venison, Milk (Low protein)

Alkaline Forming Foods	Acid Forming Foods
MISC.	**MISC.**
Butter (Sweet), Carob, Chocolate Bitter, chlorophyll, Herbal Beverage, Herb Teas, Olive Oil	Canned and prepared foods tend toward acidity. Alcohol, Artificial sweeteners, Coffee/tea, Drugs/medications, Oils (hydrogenated), Pepper, Table Salt

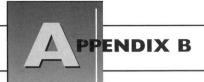

SUGGESTED READING LIST

URINE THERAPY:

THE WATER OF LIFE
by Dr. John Armstrong
A gifted healer's account of hundreds of cures through the use of natural urine therapy.

HEALING YOURSELF WITH HOMEOPATHY
by Martha M Christy
A simple, user-friendly guide for using homeopathic remedies to complement healing during urine therapy.

SIMPLE DIAGNOSTIC TESTS YOU CAN DO AT HOME
by Martha M. Christy
How to use and interpret at-home urine tests that are now commercially available for testing for conditions such as bladder and kidney infections, sugar (glucose) levels, liver function, blood in the urine, pregnancy and ovulation testing, etc. Also shows you how to detect health conditions through observing and interpreting the color and appearance of your urine.

EDUCATIONAL BOOKS

THE PROBLEMS WITH CONVENTIONAL MEDICINE:

THE BETRAYAL OF HEALTH
by Dr. Joseph Beasley
A doctor's own objective and tremendously insightful look into the reasons why modern conventional medicine has failed to cure diseases and give mankind physical and mental health and well-being. (1991)

THE INFORMED CONSUMER'S PHARMACY
by Ellen Hodgson Brown and Lynne Paige Walker
A valuable guide to understanding the real truth and side effects of synthetic drug therapy. (1990)

OVER THE COUNTER PILLS THAT DON'T WORK
by Joel Kaufman, et. al. and the Public Citizen Health Research Group,
Pantheon Books, New York. (1983)

PILLS THAT DON'T WORK
by Sidney Wolfe and Christopher M. Coley; Farrar, Strauss, and Giroux.
A consumer's guide to over 600 prescription drugs that lack evidence
of effectiveness. (1980)

MEDICINE ON TRIAL
by Charles B. Inlander, Lowell S. Levin and Ed Weiner, Prentice Hall
Press, The Appalling Story of Ineptitude, Malfeasance, Neglect and
Arrogance, (1988)

WHAT YOUR DOCTOR DIDN'T LEARN IN MEDICAL SCHOOL
And What You Can Do About It
by Stuart M Berger, M.D.

LEARNING ABOUT NATURAL MEDICINE

THE FAMILY GUIDE TO HOMEOPATHY: Symptoms and Natural
Solutions;
by Dr. Andrew Lockie; Prentice Hall Press.
One of the best introductions and guides available for using homeopathic medicines at home. (1989)

BOERICKE'S MATERIA MEDICA
The traditional guide to homeopathic remedies.

THE SCIENTIFIC VALIDATION OF HERBAL MEDICINE
by Daniel B. Mowrey; Keats Publishing, Inc.
A comprehensively researched study validating the use of natural herbs
in medicinal application. (1986)

YOUR BODY'S BEST DEFENSE: How pH Balancing Conquiers
Aging & Disease
by Martha Christy.
A simple guide to interpreting pH tests and balancing your
acid/alkaline levels.

DIET AND HEALING

HEALING WITH WHOLE FOODS
by Paul Pitchford
This comprehensive 656 page manual reads easily and is excellent for those who like a more "Westernized" approach to the macrobiotic diet. (1993)

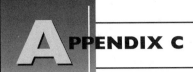

REFERENCES

Chapter Two

1. Judell, B., *"HIV Urine Testing Nearing Reality"*: **Bay Area Reporter,** August 8, 1988.

2. Burzynski, Stanislaw R., et al., *"Antineoplaston A in Cancer Therapy: Physiology,"* **Chemistry & Physics,** Vol. 9, 1977, p. 485

3. MacKay, E.M. and Schroeder, C.R.: *Virucidal (rabies and polio) activity of aqueous urea solution.* **Proceedings of the Society of Experimental Biology,** 35: 74-76, 1936.

4. Noble, R.C., et al., *"Bactericidal Properties of Urine for Neisseria gonorrhoea"*: **Sexually Transmitted Diseases.,** Vol. 14, #4, pp.221-226.

5. Wilson, C.W.M. and Lewis, A., *Auto-Immune Therapy Against Human Allergic Disease: A Physiological Self Defence Factor,* **Medical Hypotheses** 12:143 -158, 1983.

6. Myrvik, Q., Weiser, R.S., Houglum, B. and Berger, L.R.: *Studies on the Tuberculoinhibitory Properties of Ascorbic Acid Derivatives and their Possible Role in Inhibition of Tubercle Bacilli by Urine,* **The American Review of Tuberculosis,** Vol. 69 January - June 1954.

7. *"Urea: New Use of an Old Agent",* **Symposium on Surgery of the Head and Neck,** 1957.

8. Plesch, J., *"Urine-Therapy",* **Medical Press** (London), Vol.218, August 6, 1947, pp. 128-133.

9. Dunne, N.L., *The Use of Injected and Sublingual Urine in the Treatment of Allergies, A Preliminary Report,* held at Oxford Medical Symposium, 1981.

10. Hegyeli, A., .McLaughlin, J.A., and Szent-Gyorgyi, A.: *Preparation of Retine from Human Urine,* **Science,** December 20, 1963, pp. 1571-1572.

11. Smith, H., *"De Urina",* **Journal of American Medical Association,** Vol. 155, #10, pp. 899 - 902.

12. Kolata, G., *"Surgery on Fetuses Reveals They Heal Without Scars",* **New York Times,** August 16, 1988, Section C, pp. 1-3.

13. Free, A.H. and Free, H.M., **Urinalysis in Clinical Laboratory Practice,** CRC Press, Inc. 1975, pp. 13 - 17.

14. Cameron, Stewart, **Kidney Disease, The Facts,** Oxford University Press, 1986, pg. 3.

15. Staff Reporter, *"Now Urine Business,"* **Hippocrates** (Magazine), May, 1988.

16. Munk, N., *"The child is the father of the man":* **Forbes,** August 16, 1993, pp. 88 - 92.

17. **Physicians Desk Reference for Nonprescription Drugs,** Medical Economics Data Productions Co. Inc., 14th Edition, 1993.

18. **Ibid.**

19. Serup, J., *Acta Derm Venereol* (Stockholm) 1992: Suppl. 177: pp. 29 - 33.

20. Herman, J.R., *"Autourotherapy",* **New York State Journal of Medicine,** Vol. 80, #7, June, 1980, pp. 1149 - 1154.

21. Davies, O., *"Youthful Uric Acid",* **Omni Magazine** October, 1982, Continuum Section.

22. Free, A.H. and Free, H.M., **Urinalysis in Clinical And Laboratory Practice,** CRC Press, Inc. 1975, pg. 1.

Chapter Three

1. Beasley, J.D., **The Betrayal of Health,** Times Books, 1991, pp.191

2. **Ibid.**

3. Beasley, pp. 191, 194

4. **Ibid.** pp. 195,196

5. Beasley, pp. 200 - 201

6. Mowry, D.B., **The Scientific Validation of Herbal Medicine,** Keats Publishing, 1986

7. Public Citizens Health Research Group, **Over the Counter Pills That Don't Work,** Pantheon Books, 1983, pg. 10

8. Wolfe, S.M., and Coley, C.M., **Pills that Don't Work,** Farrar Straus Giroux Publishers, 1979, pg. 1.

9. Cannella, D., *"Human Guinea pig says he's lucky to be alive"*, **The Arizona Republic,** 9/2/93, pg. 1.

10. Beasley, J.D., **The Betrayal of Health,** Times Books, 1991, pg. 199.

11. Staff reporter, **The Wall Street Journal,** Jan. 11, 1994.

12. Staff Reporter, *"Factor S: Help for the Wee, Wee Hours"*, source unknown.

13. Weil, Andrew, M.D., **Health and Healing,** Houghton Mifflin Co., 1983.

14. Associated Press, *"Tuberculosis on rise in US"*, **The Arizona Republic,** 10/8/94, Section A6.

15. Phalon, R., *New support for old therapies,* **Forbes Magazine,** 12/20/1993, p.254

16. Berger, S.M., **What Your Doctor Didn't Learn in Medical School,** Wm. Morrow Publishers, 1988, pg. 16.

17. Inlander, Charles B., et. al., **Medicine On Trial, The Appalling Story of Ineptitude, Malfeasance, Neglect, and Arrogance,** Prentice Hall Press, N.Y., 1988, pp. 11-12.

18. Brown, E.H. and Walker, L.P., **The Informed Consumer's Pharmacy,** Carroll & Graf Publishers, Inc., 1990, pg.5.

19. Beasley, J.D., **The Betrayal of Health,** Times Books, 1991, pg. 201.

20. Bounds, W., *"Sick of Skyrocketing Costs, Patients Defy Doctors and Shop for Cheaper Treatment"*, **Wall Street Journal,** 6/16/93.

21. Beasley, J.D., **The Betrayal of Health,** Times Books, 1991, pg.4.

22. Giblin, P., *"Non-traditional care becoming widely accepted"*, **Focus on Behavioral Health Magazine,** Phoenix, AZ, 7/9/93, p.21

23. Friend, T., *"National health agency to study unconventional medical treatments"*, **Today Newspaper,** Melbourne, Fla., August 1993.

Chapter Four

1. Smith, H., *"De Urina"*, **Journal of American Medical Association,** Vol. 155, July 3, 1954, pp. 899 - 902.

2. Wilson, W.J.,: *"Polymorphism as exhibited by bacterial growth on media containing urea."* **J. Path. Bact.,** Lond., Vol. 11: pg. 394, 1906.

3. Spiro, Z.F., **Physiology and Chemistry,** 1900, Vol. 30, p. 182.

4. Ramsden, W., *"Some new properties of Urea"*, **The Proceedings of the Physiological Society,** July 5, 1902, pg. xxiii.

5. Peju, G., and Rajat, H., *"Note sur le polymorphisme des bacteries dans l'uree,* **Compt. rend. Soc. de Biol.,** Volume 61: pg. 477, 1906.

6. Symmers, W.S.C., and Kirk, T.S., *"Urea as a bactericide and its applications in the treatment of wounds"*, **Lancet Volume** 2: pp. 1237, 1915

7. Duncan, C.H., **Autotherapy,** New York: C.H. Duncan, 1918.

8. Millar, W.M., *"Urea Crystals in Cancer"* **Journ. A.M.A.,** May 27, 1933, pg. 1684.

9. Krebs, M., *"Auto-Urine Therapy"*, **Society of Pediatricians,** Leipzig, 1934, p. 442 - 444.

10. Tiberi, R., *"Value of Auto-Uro-Vaccine Therapy in Acute Hemorrhagic Nephritis"*, **La Diagnosi,** Vol. 14, 6/9/34, pp. 183 - 196.

11. Mckay, E.M., and Schroeder, C.R., *"Virucidal (rabies and polio) activity of aqueous urea solution"*, **Proc. Soc. Exper. Biol.,** 35: 74-76, 1936.

12. Muldavin, L., and Holtsman, J.M., *"Treatment of Infected Wounds with Urea"*, **The Lancet,** March 3, 1938, pg. 549.

13. Sandweiss, D.J., Sugarman, M.H., Friedman, M.H.F., and Saltzstein, H.C., *"The Effect of Urine Extracts on Peptic Ulcer"*, **Journ. D.D.,** Oct. 1941, pp. 371 - 382.

14. Armstrong, J., **The Water of Life,** C.W. Daniel Publishers, 1944.

15. Weinstein, L. and McDonald, A.: *The action of urea and some of its derivatives on bacteria,* **Journal of Immunology,** Volume 54: pp. 117 - 149, 1946.

16. *"Fourth Annual Report on Carcinogens"*, **Journal of Advanced Cancer Research,** 1986.

17. Plesch, J., *"Urine-Therapy"*, **Medical Press** (London), Vol. 218, August 6, 1947, pp. 371 - 382.

18. Bjornesjo, K.B., *"On the Effect of Human Urine on Tubercle Bacilli II: The Tuberculostatic Effect on Various Urine Constituents"*, **Acta Scandinavica,** Vol. 25, No.5, 1951, pp. 447-455.

19. Myrvik, Q., et al., *"Studies on the Tuberculoinhibitory Properties of Ascorbic Acid Derivatives and Their Possible Role in Inhibition of Tubercle Bacilli by Urine"*, **American Review of Tuberculosis,** Vol. 69, No.3, March 1954, pp. 406 - 418.

20. Tsuji, S., et al., *"Isolation from Human Urine of a Polypeptide Having Marked Tuberculostatic Activity"*, **American Review of Respiratory Diseases,** Vol. 91, No. 6, June 1965, pp. 832-838.

21. Associate Press, *"Tuberculosis on rise in US"*, **Arizona Republic,** 10/8/93, Section A 6.

22. Tsuji, S., Ibid #20.

23. Lerner, A.M., et al., *"Neutralizing Antibody to Polioviruses in Normal Human Urine"*, **Journal of Clinical Investigation,** Vol. 41, No. 4, April, 1962, pp. 805-815.

24. Dunne, M.P., *"The Use of Injected and Sublingual Urine in the Treatment of Allergies"*, *A Preliminary Report,* held at the Oxford Medical Symposium, 1981.

25. Kaye, Donald, *"Antibacterial Activity of Human Urine"*, **Journal of Clinical Investigation,** Vol. 47, 1968, pp. 2374-90.

26. Dunne, N.P., **Ibid** #24.

27. *"Effect of Urea on Cerebrospinal Fluid Pressure in Human Subjects"*, **Journal of the American Medical Association,** Vol. 160, No. 11, 3/17/56, pp. 943 - 949.

28. **Ibid.**

29. *"Urea: New Use of an Old Agent"*, **Symposium on Surgery of the Head and Neck,** 1957.

30. **Physicians Desk Reference,** 1992, page 1200.

31. Schlegel, J.U., Cueller, J., and O'Dell, R.M., *"Bactericidal Effect of Urea"*, **The Journal of Urology,** Vol. 86, No.6, Dec. 1961, pp.819-822.

32. Free and Free, A.H., and H.M., **Urinalysis in Clinical and Laboratory Practice,** Chapter 1, pg. 13.

33. **Handbook of Toxic and Hazardous Chemicals and Carcinogens,** 1985.

34. Kaye, D., *"Antibacterial Activity of Human Urine"*, **Journal of Clinical Investigation,** Vol. 47, 1968, pp. 2374 - 2390.

35. Lerner, A.M., et al., *"Neutralizing Antibody to Polioviruses in Normal Human Urine"*, **Journal of Clinical Investigation,** Vol. 41, No. 4, April, 1962, pp. 805-815.

36. Berger, R., et al., *"Demonstration of IgA Polioantibody in Saliva, Duodenal fluid and Urine"*, **Nature,** Vol. 214, April 22, 1967, pp. 420-422.

37. Giordano, C., *"The Use of Exogenous and Endogenous Urea for Protein Synthesis in Normal and Uremic Subjects"*, **Renal Laboratory,** Naples University School of Medicine, 1963.

38. Hanson, Lars A., et al., *"Characterization of Antibodies in Human Urine"*, **Journal of Clinical Investigation,** Vol. 44, No. 5, 1965, pp. 703 - 715.

39. Free and Free, **Urinalysis in Clinical and Laboratory Practice,** pg. 32.

40. Szent-Gyorgi, et al., *"Preparation of Retine from Human Urine"*, **Science,** Dec. 30, 1963, pp. 1571 - 1572.

41. Soeda, Momoe, *"Treatment of Gastric Cancer with HUD, an Antigenic Substance obtained from Patient's Urine"*, **Tokyo Nihon Igaku Hoshasen Gakkai,** Vol. 28, 12/25/68, pp. 1265 - 1278.

42. **Ibid.**

43. Burzynski, S.R., et al., *"Antineoplaston A in Cancer Therapy"*, **Physiology, Chemistry, & Physics,** Vol. 9, 1977, pg. 485.

44. Null, Gary, *"The Suppression of Cancer Cures"*, **Penthouse,** Oct. 1979, pp. 90 - 95.

45. Beasley, **The Betrayal of Health,** 1993, Times Books, p. 206.

46. Armstrong, J., **The Water of Life.**

47. Beasley, **The Betrayal of Health,** 1993, Times Books, p.206.

48. McMenamin, B., *"An educated consumer is the best patient"*, **Forbes,** June 21, 1993, pg. 118.

49. Kent, S., *"DHEA: Miracle Drug?"*, **Geriatics,** Vol. 37, No. 9, 1982, pp. 157 - 161.

50. Celia Farber, *A.I.D.S. Words From the Front,* **Co-Factors Magazine,** June, 1988, pg. 81, 82.

51. Farber, C., and Lederer, B., *"AIDS, Words From the Front"*, **Spin Magazine** Vol. 5, No.3, June 1989, pp.90-107.

52. Staff Reporter, *"HIV Urine Testing Nearing Reality"* **Bay Area Reporter,** August 8, 1990, pg. 1.

53. International Immunology Institute, **"Immuno-Tolerance"**, Physician's Handbook, 1982 pp. 1, 16.

54. **Ibid.,** pp.1, 16.

55. Dunne, N.P., *"The Use of Injected and Sublingual Urine in the Treatment of Allergies"*, A Preliminary Report held at Oxford Medical Symposium, 1981.

56. International Immunology Institute, *"Immuno-Tolerance"*, **Physicians's Handbook,** 1982, pp. 1, 16.

57. Linscott, William D., **Specific Immunologic Unresponsiveness, Basic and Clinical Immunology,** Lange Medical Publications, 3rd Edition, 1982.

58. Wilson, C.W.M., and Lewis, A., *"Auto-Immune Therapy Against Human Allergic Disease: A Physiological Self Defense Factor"*, **Medical Hypothesis,** Vol. 12, 1983, p. 143.

59. Wilson, C.W.M., *"The Protective Effect of Auto-Immune Buccal Urine Therapy (AIBUT) Against the Raynaud Phenomenon"*, Medical **Hypothesis,** Vol. 13: 99-107, 1984.

60. Noble, R.C., et al., *"Bactericidal Properties of Urine for Nesseria gonorrhoeae"*, **Sexually Transmitted Diseases,** Vol.14, #4, Oct-Dec 1987, pp. 221-226.

61. Liao, Z., et al., *"Identification of a Specific Interleukin 1 Inhibitor in the Urine of Febrile Patients"*, **Journal of Experimental Medicine,** Rockefeller University Press, Vol. 159, January, 1984, pp. 126 - 136.

63. Mannucci, P.M. and D'Angelo, A., *Urokinase, Basic and Clinical Aspects,* **Serono Symposia.** Academic Press, 1982.

64. Staff Writers, *"Blood Clots: Legs and Lungs"*, **Harvard Medical School Health Letter,** Vol. 10, No. 3, January, 1985. pg.5.

65. Swanbeck, G., *"Urea in the Treatment of Dry Skin"*, **Acta Derm Venereol** (Stockholm), 1992; Suppl. 177: pp. 7-8.

66. Serup, J., *"A Double-blind Comparison of Two Creams Containing Urea as the Active Ingredient"*, **Acta Derm Venereol** (Stockholm), 1992; Suppl. 177: pp. 34-38.

67. Ibid.

68. **Physician's Desk Reference for Non-Prescription Drugs,** Medical Economics Data Production, 1993.

69. Decaux, G., et al., *"Five Year Treatment of the Chronic Syndrome of Inappropriate Secretion of ADH with Oral Urea"*, **Nephron** 1993; Vol. 63: pp. 468-470.

Chapter Five

1. Smith, H., *"De Urina"*, **Journal of American Medical Association,** Vol. 155, July 3, 1954, pp. 899 - 902.

2. Herman, J.R., *"Autourotherapy"*, **New York State Journal of Medicine,** Vol. 80, #7, June, 1980, pp. 1149 - 1154.

3. Smith, Homer, **Ibid #1**

4. Wallnufer, Heinrich, **Chinese Folk Medicine and Acupuncture,** Crown Publishers, N.Y., p.71

5. Shankardevananda, Dr. S., **Amaroli,** Bihar School, 1978, pp. 8-9.

6. Patel, Raojibhai, **Manav Mootra (Auto-Urine Therapy),** Bharat Sevak Samj Publications, Pankornaka, India, 1973.

INDEX

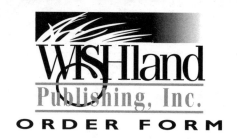

WISHland
Publishing, Inc.
O R D E R   F O R M

Name _____ Phone _____

Address _____

City _____ State _____ Zip _____

Qty.	Item #	Description	Cost	Total
	W1500	Your Own Perfect Medicine by Martha Christy	$19.95	
	W1516	The Golden Fountain by Coen van der Kroon	15.95	
	W1501	The Water of Life by John Armstrong	11.95	
	W1900	Simple Diagnostic Tests You can Do At Home by Martha Christy	11.95	
	W1379	On The Track Of Water's Secret by H. Kronberger & S. Lattacher	14.95	
	W1902	Chemstrips Screening Test (10 Strips)	15.99	
	W1907	pH Monitoring Roll	11.95	
	W1505	PureaSkin Unscented Lotion	9.95	
	W1507	PureaSkin Unscented Cream	11.95	
	W1502	Scientific Validation of Urine Therapy by Martha Christy	11.00	
	W1503	You're in Good Health: 22 Testimonials of self-healing with urine therapy	11.00	
	W1504	Urine Therapy Introduction: Bruce Holmes Interviews Martha Christy	11.00	
	W1512	How To Fast On Urine Therapy	15.00	
	W1513	101 Ways To Use Urine Therapy	11.00	
	W1509	USP Grade Urea Crystals (1 lb.)	19.50	

Shipping & Handling
1 - 3 Items $ 4.00
4 + Items $ 8.00
10 + Items $10.00
Next Day Service Available.

Foreign Orders, ADD $35.00 to charges, orders to Canada add $25.00.

Arizona residents only - ADD 7.4% TAX

TOTAL AMOUNT ENCLOSED

Make checks payable to *Wishland, Inc.*
For Credit Card orders, call **1-800-559-2873**   ❏ Visa   ❏ MC   ❏ Discover   ❏ Am Ex

Acct. # _____ Exp. Date _____

Signature_____ Date _____

Send Order to: Wishland, Inc.,   P.O. Box 41504, Mesa, AZ 85274
(480) 922-8511   Fax: (480) 443-3386   To Order: 1-800-559-2873